Complete Guide to Carb Counting

2nd edition

Hope S. Warshaw, MMSc, RD, CDE, BC-ADM
Karmeen Kulkarni, MS, RD, CDE, BC-ADM

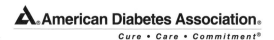

American Diabetes Association®

Cure • Care • Commitment®

Director, Book Publishing, John Fedor; *Associate Director, Consumer Books,* Sherrye Landrum; *Editor,* Abe Ogden; *Associate Director, Book Production,* Peggy M. Rote; *Composition,* Circle Graphics; *Cover Design,* Koncept, Inc.; *Printer,* Worzalla.

Printed in the United States of America
3 5 7 9 10 8 6 4 2

The suggestions and information contained in this publication are generally consistent with the *Clinical Practice Recommendations* and other policies of the American Diabetes Association, but they do not represent the policy or position of the Association or any of its boards or committees. Reasonable steps have been taken to ensure the accuracy of the information presented. However, the American Diabetes Association cannot ensure the safety or efficacy of any product or service described in this publication. Individuals are advised to consult a physician or other appropriate health care professional before undertaking any diet or exercise program or taking any medication referred to in this publication. Professionals must use and apply their own professional judgment, experience, and training and should not rely solely on the information contained in this publication before prescribing any diet, exercise, or medication. The American Diabetes Association—its officers, directors, employees, volunteers, and members—assumes no responsibility or liability for personal or other injury, loss, or damage that may result from the suggestions or information in this publication.

⊚ The paper in this publication meets the requirements of the ANSI Standard Z39.48-1992 (permanence of paper).

ADA titles may be purchased for business or promotional use or for special sales. To purchase this book in large quantities, or for custom editions of this book with your logo, contact Lee Romano Sequeira, Special Sales & Promotions, at the address below, or at LRomano@diabetes.org or 703-299-2046.

American Diabetes Association
1701 North Beauregard Street
Alexandria, Virginia 22311

Library of Congress Cataloging-in-Publication Data
Warshaw, Hope S., 1954-
    Complete guide to carb counting / Hope S. Warshaw, Karmeen Kulkarni.—2nd ed.
    p. cm.
    Includes index.
    ISBN 1-58040-203-8 (pbk. : alk. Paper)
    1. Diabetes—Diet therapy. 2. Food—Carbohydrate content. I. Kulkarni, Karmeen, 1953-   II. Title.

RC662.W313 2004
616.4'620654—dc22

2004050918

*This book is dedicated to all people with diabetes.
We hope it provides you with the
knowledge and skills to
make carb counting a central part of
your diabetes care and
helps you to achieve the diabetes control and
quality of life that you desire.*

Contents

Foreword

Carbohydrates (or more precisely, lack thereof) have been receiving a lot of attention lately. It seems that with the growing popularity of the various low-carbohydrate diets now flooding the market (diets, it should be noted, that have not been backed by serious scientific evidence) it's nearly impossible to visit a grocery store, eat at a restaurant, or even open a newspaper without hearing about carbs. For those with diabetes, attention to carbohydrate is nothing new. Even before the discovery of insulin, the early diets severely restricted carbohydrate intake. Over time, our understanding of carbohydrates improved. As the decades passed and research continued it became clear that carbohydrates had the largest impact on blood glucose levels. Eventually, it was shown that not only sugar had this effect, but all carbohydrates. By the turn of the century, one of the main challenges of diabetes therapy was to match carbohydrate content to insulin availability (whether made by your body or injected from outside).

Just from a conceptual point of view, this notion seems easy enough to understand. However, as anyone who has ever tried to put this theory into practice appreciates, the process can be exceedingly difficult. Immediately a host of questions spring to mind: What is a carbohydrate? What foods contain carbohydrate? How much carbohydrate should a person eat? How do you count all of this carbohydrate? And perhaps ultimately, how does this help diabetes management? Suddenly, what at first seemed like a simple matter of adding numbers can become overwhelming.

Fortunately, this is a good time to be a "carb counter." There are a variety of resources available to help you in your pursuit of counted carbohydrates. Nutrition information detailing the amount of carbohydrate in foods is widely available, whether it is printed on the Nutrition Facts label on packaged food products, available in a brochure at a restaurant, listed on a website, or catalogued in a carb count book. Many cookbooks, including all of those from the American Diabetes Association, list the nutrition information for their recipes. Weights and measuring devices, essential pieces of Advanced Carbohydrate Counting, can be easily ordered from websites. In other words, the tools and aids available to you as a burgeoning Carb Counter are almost unlimited. Unfortunately, these types of tools are often under-utilized. Recent studies have shown that the majority of people who count their carbohydrates misestimate what they are actually eating. The reason for this, in my view, is not that the tools and aids are ineffective, but rather they are not used effectively.

Furthermore, tools and aids can only do so much. They are not a method. Just because you have a hammer and saw doesn't mean you can build a house. To move forward you need a clear and cohesive blueprint. To build a strong Carb Counting program, think of this book as your blueprint. Within these pages, the authors provide a simple, easy-to-follow Carb Counting plan that can be tailored to any diabetes management regimen. They teach you how carbohydrates affect your blood glucose, how to use the tools available to you, why different carbohydrates act differently in your body, and much more. They provide tips and tricks to make the process easier. And they present all of this information in a clear, easy-to-understand format that makes the process of learning as simple as possible.

As I mentioned above, people new to Carb Counting often find they have a lot of questions. However, all of these can be distilled down to two basic questions that form the foundation for the rest: Why should I count carbohydrates? And how do I count carbohydrates? The answers to both can be found in this book, which should be read by every physician, educator, and individual with diabetes.

Irl B. Hirsch, MD
June, 2004
Seattle, WA

Acknowledgments

Thanks to several colleagues who provided valuable critiques: Sandy Gillespie, MMSc, RD, CDE, and David Shade, MD. Thanks to Anne Daly, MS, RD, CDE, for reviewing the manuscript and Irl Hirsch, MD, for writing the Foreword. Thanks to Virginia Valentine, MS, RD, CDE; Ginger Kanzer Lewis, MS, RD, CDE; and Nicole Johnson for their review and quotes. The authors also thank J. Scott Rainey, a patient with type 1 diabetes, for his thorough review and thoughtful comments.

Thanks to the staff at ADA—Sherrye, Peggy, Keith, and Lee—who helped to edit and prepare the manuscript for printing and developed marketing and publicity to ensure the success of this book.

1

Why Count Carbs?

Would you like to have a better sense of when your blood glucose is going to rise, and more than that, about how high it might go today, tomorrow, or the next day? If your answer is YES, then the approach to planning your meals called Carbohydrate Counting—Carb Counting for short—might be just what you need to gain better control of your blood glucose levels.

Foods contain varying amounts of carbohydrate, protein, fat, vitamins, minerals, and water. When you use Carb Counting you only need to pay attention to the carbohydrate in food. But how can that be? It's because it is the carbohydrate in foods that raises your blood glucose the quickest and the most. Simply put, count the carbohydrate in the cereal, banana, and milk that you ate for breakfast, and check how high your blood glucose is one to two hours later. The next morning you eat the same amount of carbohydrate as you did the day before, only in different foods. And lo and behold, when you check one to two hours later, your blood glucose is around the same level as it was yesterday! The first two mornings you don't do any exercise, but you do take your diabetes medication. The third morning after you eat the same cereal and banana breakfast you had the first day, you take a walk. Surprise! Your blood glucose level one to two hours later is lower than it was on the other days. That's evidence that carbs raise your blood glucose and physical activity lowers it.

To make things easier, you could just choose to eat cereal with milk and banana for breakfast every day and find that your blood glucose levels fall into a predictable pattern. But who wants, or is even willing, to eat the same meal 365 days a year? No one! Tomorrow you may want a waffle, a half of a grapefruit, and bacon. The next day you might be on the road and choose an Egg McMuffin and orange juice. With Carb Counting, you can feel comfortable changing your food choices day to day!

Variety: The Spice of Life

Just because you have diabetes doesn't mean you have to eat a limited scope of foods. With an understanding of Carb Counting, you can enjoy a wide variety of American foods, foods from your culture, and foods from a variety of cultures; as long as you can and do count the carbs you eat. You can add new foods to your breakfast, lunch, and dinner selections without risking unexpected high blood glucose levels. Consistency is the key to Carb Counting. If you eat about the same amount of carbohydrate at each meal and snack each day, your blood glucose levels are more likely to fall into a steady pattern, which means better diabetes control for you. You CAN take the mystery out of some of the ups and downs of your blood glucose.

Carb Counting May Not Be Right for Everyone

Before you jump right in, you should consider whether Carb Counting is the right approach to eating for you. Carb Counting is an approach that is being taught to many people with diabetes and it can be used by people with all types of diabetes, from type 2 to type 1 and even for women with gestational diabetes. But, it's by no means the only approach you can learn and apply.

One aspect of Carb Counting that makes it so attractive is its flexibility, not only in terms of your meal planning, but also within the system itself. Carb Counting can be simplified—known as Basic Carb Counting—or you can progress, if need be, to Advanced Carb Counting. Generally, Basic Carbohydrate Counting works well if you have type 2 diabetes and control it with a healthy eating plan and physical activity with or without the addition of oral diabetes medications. Basic Carb Counting is also a good starting point if you have type 2 and take one type of insulin or a combination of insulin and oral diabetes medications. However, if you have type 1 or type 2 diabetes and you take several shots (three to four) of insulin a day or use an insulin pump, you'll likely want to progress to Advanced Carbohydrate Counting. This provides you with a lot more flexibility—the ability to adjust the amount of rapid-acting insulin you take and carb you eat, as well as when you eat.

As you learn more about Carb Counting in the pages ahead, ask yourself whether you think this approach will fit your needs and lifestyle. In chapter 3 you'll get to do a self-assessment to determine if Carb Counting is right for you. You'll also get a chance in chapter 12 to do another self-assessment to determine if you want or need to progress from Basic to Advanced Carb Counting.

Now, let's get into Carb Counting by first learning which foods contain carbohydrate.

WHICH FOODS CONTAIN CARBOHYDRATE?

You probably answered starches, such as potatoes and corn. Then you add bread, cereal, rice, crackers, and pasta. Oh, and don't forget the starchy vegetables—peas, beans, and lentils. If you're like most people, that's where you stop. That's because people tend to equate carbohydrates with starches. Starches, such as all those mentioned above, contain carbohydrate, but other foods also fall under the "carbohydrate umbrella." Here is a complete list of the food groups whose foods contain calories mainly from carbohydrate:

- Starches—bread, cereal, crackers, rice, pasta, potatoes, and corn

- Starchy vegetables—peas, beans, and lentils

- Fruit and fruit juice

- Vegetables—nonstarchy, such as green beans, lettuce, and carrots (Note: Though these contain carbohydrate, they contain small amounts. To get all the desirable vitamins and minerals, most people need to eat more vegetables.)

- Milk, yogurt, and other dairy foods (Note: the amount of carb in dairy foods varies quite a bit. On average, 8 ounces (oz) of most cheese contains about 8 grams (g) of carb, yet 8 oz of milk contains 12 g of carb. Learn the amount of carb in dairy foods by checking the Nutrition Facts label.)

- Sugary foods, such as candy (gum drops, jelly beans), regular soda, fruit punch, and sports drinks

- Sweets, such as candy (chocolate bars), cakes, cookies, and pies

Once you read this list you might scratch your head wondering which foods *do not* contain carbohydrate. That list is shorter—meats (red meat, poultry, seafood, and eggs) and fats (oil, butter, bacon, and nuts). But, just because these foods don't contain carbohydrate doesn't mean you don't have to pay some attention to the types and amounts of them you eat. They contain calories and there are certainly some meat choices that are healthier than others. You can learn more about protein and fats in chapter 6.

HOW MUCH CARBOHYDRATE IS IN IT?

Table 1-1 lists average amounts of carbohydrate in some general food groups. This table helps you start to learn how much carb is

TABLE 1-1	Nutrients			
Food group	**Serving***	**Carbohydrate (g)**	**Protein (g)**	**Fat (g)**
Bread	1 slice	15	3	0
Cereal, dry	1 oz	15	3	†
Cereal, cooked	1/2 cup	15	3	†
Pasta, cooked	1/3 cup	15	3	†
Starchy vegetable	1/3 to 1/2 cup	15	3	0
Fruit, fresh	1 small, 1/2 large	15	0	0
Fruit, canned, no sugar added	1/2 cup	15	0	0
Vegetables, cooked	1/2 cup	5	0	0
Vegetables, raw	1 cup	5	0	0
Milk, fat free	1 cup	12	8	0
Yogurt, plain, fat-free	2/3 cup	12	8	0
Sugary foods	1 serving	Varies	Varies	Varies
Sweets	1 serving	Varies	Varies	Varies
Meats	3 oz cooked	0	21	Varies
Fats— margarine, mayonnaise, oil	1 tsp	0	0	5

* Servings are from *Exchange Lists for Meal Planning* published by ADA and The American Dietetic Association, 2003.
† Depends on the product.

in various categories of foods. Check to see how much carb are in a typical slice of commercial bread—15 g of carbohydrate. In "Appendix 1. Carb Counts of Everyday Foods," we expand this list by many fold. It provides the exact amount of carbohydrate in five hundred foods Americans most commonly eat. Then, to expand your horizons even further, "Appendix 2. Carb Counting

Resources," gives you a list of books and other resources where you can find the amount of carbohydrate in nearly any food you can think of—from apples to zabaglione. If you are going to follow Carb Counting, it's important for you to have some resources—especially if you eat foods that don't have Nutrition Facts labels, such as fresh fruit and vegetables or restaurant foods.

HOW DOES CARB COUNTING HELP WITH BLOOD GLUCOSE CONTROL?

You can count the carbs in every food you eat for the rest of your life, but unless you make some notes about how they affect your blood glucose level, you won't have the information you need. What's on your fork? Write it down. What's your blood glucose? Write it down. The first few weeks of Carb Counting are the science experiment—perhaps one of the most important ones you'll ever do. With Carb Counting, curiosity, data collection, and analysis definitely pay off. Chapter 11 helps you learn what you need to record and how to analyze your results.

WHAT'S SO IMPORTANT ABOUT CONTROLLING YOUR BLOOD GLUCOSE LEVELS?

When you keep your blood glucose levels near normal, you feel better today and tomorrow. You also help prevent and/or delay long-term complications of diabetes, such as eye, heart, and kidney problems. Think of keeping your blood glucose levels in control like walking on a balance beam—you don't want to fall off on either side. You don't want your blood glucose too high or too low too often.

Table 1-2, Target Ranges for Blood Glucose and A1C Levels, gives you the blood glucose levels that the American Diabetes Association (ADA) recommends. Discuss with your health care provider what your target levels should be. Yours may be different from the ones in the table for a variety of reasons. For example, a pregnant woman may have lower target levels and an older

TABLE 1-2 Target Ranges for Blood Glucose and A1C Levels	
Test	**Goal**
Average fasting and premeal blood glucose	90–130 mg/dl (plasma)
Average postmeal blood glucose level (1–2 hours after the start of a meal)	<180 mg/dl (plasma)
A1C (%)	<7% (normal range is based on 4–6%)

person at risk for hypoglycemia may have higher target levels than those in Table 1-2. In general, if you keep your blood glucose levels and A1C (the three-month average of your blood glucose levels) in the target ranges, you have the best chance at feeling good today and staying as healthy as possible for the rest of your life.

Basic Facts about Carbohydrate

All the carbohydrate you eat is broken down into glucose (sugar) by about two hours from the time you start to eat. Carbohydrates are the body's main and preferred energy source. There are three categories of carbohydrates: starches, sugars, and fibers. Starches and sugars are the main contributors of carbohydrate to our foods. Fiber is carbohydrate, but depending on the type—soluble or insoluble—its impact on blood glucose differs.

The terms or categories of simple and complex carbohydrates that were used for many years are no longer used because research suggests that these terms don't sufficiently explain how the various types of carbohydrates affect blood glucose. In fact, it can't be assumed that sugar or juice, for example, raises blood glucose faster than some starches. Sometimes the converse is true.

Once you eat any type of carb, it is broken down into glucose that goes into your bloodstream. With the help of the hormone insulin, the cells of your body can use the glucose in your blood for energy. At this point, your body doesn't know whether the glucose came from the carbohydrate in mashed potatoes or a piece of apple pie. All carbohydrates become glucose—the body's favorite source of energy.

IF CARBS RAISE BLOOD GLUCOSE, SHOULD YOU FOLLOW A LOW-CARB DIET?

Once you realize that carbohydrates raise blood glucose, you might jump to the conclusion that, if you have diabetes, it's best to steer clear of them. And that certainly might be your conclusion if you read up on one of the low-carb diet regimens. These diets sound like they are made-to-order for people with type 2 diabetes. The reality is that at this point, the science to support the long-term use of low-carb diets (less than 40% of calories as carbohydrate) for long-term weight loss and maintenance simply doesn't exist. Just a handful of well-done studies have been conducted since 2000. Though these are solid research studies, they're relatively short—just six months to one year.

What these studies show about weight loss with low-carb diets:

- Some studies show that people lost a few more pounds on low carb and high protein than the converse. Yet other studies don't show much difference, especially when the studies last a year.

- A low-carb diet doesn't cause a worsening of blood lipid levels, and initially may reduce lipids, but they don't show much greater improvement of lipids than a moderate-carb eating plan or a long term loss.

- A lower- (not necessarily low-) carb eating plan (about 40%) may be more beneficial than a moderate-carb plan (45–50%) to help people lower their triglycerides. (People with type 2 diabetes, especially when first diagnosed, tend to have high triglycerides.) Both options are provided in Table 2-3 in chapter 2.

What the studies on low-carb diets show about long-term weight maintenance:

- The long-term effectiveness of low-carb eating plans hasn't been proven. That's in part because the long-term studies have never been done. Several studies are underway at reputable institutions. At this point many diabetes experts conclude that there's insufficient evidence to recommend low-carb diets, especially to people with type 2 diabetes. Beyond the question of long-term effectiveness, there are safety concerns about their long-term use, such as about the progression of heart and kidney problems.

The best advice? Find a sensible and realistic healthy eating plan for you that is based on sound science. The eating plan should help you lose weight (if you need to) and, even more importantly, keep it off the rest of your life.

A few pointers about carbohydrate:

- Don't skimp on the healthier carbohydrates. These foods are among the healthiest foods to eat. Most of the carbohydrate you eat should come from fruits, vegetables, whole grains, and low-fat dairy foods. These foods give you your biggest nutrition bang for your calorie buck. They also contain essential vitamins and minerals you don't get in other foods. You need to eat them to be healthy.

- From the group of healthy carbs, choose foods that contain fiber—whole grains, fruits, and vegetables.

- Do skimp on the not-so-healthy carbs—sugars and sweets. Eat a minimal amount of these foods. They can contribute concentrated amounts of calories and fats and add little in the way of essential vitamins and minerals. Skimp on these not because they raise blood glucose faster, which they don't, but because they simply don't offer much in the way of health.

WHAT'S LOW, MODERATE, AND HIGH?

The terms "low carb" and "high carb" get thrown around without much definition attached. For your frame of reference, it's important to know that food consumption studies from the last few years show that Americans eat about 50% of their calories in the form of carb. That's moderate carb, not high carb. So what's all the fuss about "too much" carbohydrate? The reality is that the discussion should be focused more on quality versus quantity. Americans today eat too much not-so-healthy carb—sweets, regularly sweetened drinks, and refined starches—and too little healthier carb, such as whole grains, unrefined starches, fruits, vegetables, and low-fat dairy foods.

And moderate carb from the above mentioned healthy carbs is what the American Diabetes Association recommends for most people with diabetes—roughly 45–50%. That's not high carb. The American Diabetes Association recommends that if you've had a hard time losing weight and your triglycerides are high, you might have more success by eating 40% of your calories from carb. But, do remember to keep the saturated fat low and to use more healthier fats.

WHAT ABOUT SUGARS?

First, let's get a few facts straight. Note the plural on "sugars" in the header above. The sources of sugars in our diet are way more than just the white granular stuff. There are sugars that occur naturally in foods, such as the fructose in fruit and the lactose in milk. Other sugars—such as high-fructose corn syrup—are added to foods when they are processed. From the current Nutrition Facts label on our foods, it's impossible to distinguish under "sugars," which is under Total Carbohydrates, whether these are sugars that occur naturally in the foods or if they are added sugars.

The most important thing to remember about sugars is that they are carbohydrate and will raise your blood glucose. When you eat any of the following, remember they contain carbohydrate:

- Sweeteners you find in your pantry—granulated sugar, brown sugar, honey, maple syrup—and the sweeteners used in commercial food products that you see on the food label—high-fructose corn syrup, corn sweeteners, and dextrose

- Sugary foods, such as regular soda, candy, jelly, and sweetened fruit drinks

- Sweets, such as cake, cookies, pie, chocolate candy, and desserts. Sweets usually also contain fat—and lots of calories—but for Carb Counting we focus on the carbohydrates that will raise your blood glucose level.

IF I HAVE DIABETES, CAN I EAT SUGARY FOODS AND SWEETS?

Throughout the 20th century, the most widely held belief about diabetes meal planning was to "avoid sugar." However, in the past twenty years, little scientific evidence has been found to support this notion. In fact, fruits and milk have been shown to have a lower effect on blood glucose than bread, potatoes, or beans. Table sugar has about the same effect on blood glucose that bread, rice, and potatoes do. So, now we know that what's most important for controlling your blood glucose level is the **total amount of carbohydrate in the meal—not the type of carbohydrate you eat.** This is a hard concept for a lot of people and you may need to educate your family and friends about this "new" thinking about sugars, sweets, and diabetes. People continue to believe that if you have diabetes, sugars and sweets are strictly forbidden.

So, you *can* eat sugars and sweets. But (and this is a big "but") you will need to substitute these sugars and sweets into your eating plan for other carbohydrates or adjust your diabetes medications to account for the extra carbohydrate. This may be a difficult concept for people with diabetes to accept (or for your friends and family). Are we saying that you can eat all the desserts you want? No! Nor are we suggesting that you have sweets every day. We are suggesting, however, that you learn how to work sweets into your eating plan based on your health and nutrition needs and goals, as well as your desires.

If you simply are not a sweets eater, then continue to steer clear of them. If, on the other hand, you can't live without them, go ahead and enjoy them once in a while. Here are the ADA's general guidelines for eating sugary foods and sweets:

- Substitute sugary foods or sweets for other carbohydrates in your meal plan.

- If you choose to eat a sweet, then lighten up on other carbohydrates in the meal—for example, have smaller or fewer servings of bread, potato, or fruit.

- Burn the extra calories from sweets with more exercise. (How long do you need to walk to balance the effects of that doughnut?)

Also keep in mind the following points to help you decide how often to eat sugary foods and sweets:

- Limit sugary and sweet foods until you get your blood glucose and A1C under control.

- If one of your goals is to lose some weight, then you'll need to keep sweets to a once-in-a-while frequency. Too many sweets equal too many calories.

- If your total cholesterol, LDL, HDL, and triglycerides are out of control, we recommend that you keep sweets to a minimum. Get your blood fats close to normal before you add more sweets to your meal plan (see chapter 6).

- What triggers you to want to eat sweets? Think about how much you enjoy sweets and how often you want to eat them. Can you use this information to create realistic diabetes, nutrition, and health goals?

Fiber and Blood Glucose

The fiber in foods, called dietary fiber, is another source of carbohydrate. The main sources of fiber are foods that contain most of their calories from carbohydrate—whole grains, breads, cereals, beans and peas, and fruits and vegetables. Fiber can affect how quickly your food is digested and, if eaten in very large quantities, can have an effect on your blood glucose level as well. Some research shows that a very high-fiber diet can also improve total and LDL cholesterol. The reality is that most Americans don't eat nearly the amount of fiber we need, let alone the amount needed to improve blood glucose and lipids. On average, Americans eat about 10–13 g of dietary fiber per day. The U.S. Government nutrition recommendations suggest you get 20–35 g of dietary fiber per day—just about double what most of us get.

There are two types of dietary fiber—insoluble and soluble.

- **Insoluble fibers** give form to foods. Foods that contain insoluble fiber are whole-grain cereals and breads. Insoluble fibers grab onto liquid as they travel down the gastrointestinal tract. That's good because the combination of fiber and liquid pushes food through the gastrointestinal tract more quickly. If you eat a good supply of insoluble fiber to promote a bulkier and softer bowel movement, you also reap other health benefits—preventing hemorrhoids, diverticulosis, and colon and rectal cancer.

- **Soluble fibers** dissolve during digestion but remain gummy and thick. Food sources of soluble fiber are beans, peas, and some grains, such as oats and barley. The benefits of soluble fiber are different from insoluble fibers. The soluble fibers can prevent the body from absorbing certain nutrients in foods. Two important ones are cholesterol and glucose. It is thought that eating a lot of soluble fiber can lower blood cholesterol a small amount by binding onto it during digestion. It is also thought that eating a lot of soluble fiber can lower the rise of blood glucose by slowing down the absorption of glucose.

Easy Tips to Fit in Fiber

- Choose whole-grain cereals. Use whole grains for starches, such as barley, bulgur, and buckwheat. Use more beans and peas.

- Choose fruits and vegetables high in fiber, such as acorn and butternut squash, greens, berries, and dried fruit.

- Look for whole-grain breads, cereals, and crackers, which are an "excellent" or "good" source of fiber. The U.S. Food and Drug Administration (FDA) defines "excellent" as more that 5 g per serving and "good" as between 2.5 and 4.9 g per serving.

What Is the Glycemic Index and Should I Use It with Carb Counting?

The glycemic index is a list of foods and how they affect blood glucose levels. It was developed in the early 1980s by researchers who studied how quickly or slowly various carbohydrate-containing foods raised blood glucose—bread, corn, pasta, beans, fruit, and others. The glycemic index research helped to show that not all carbohydrates raise blood glucose levels the same amount. They showed, for instance, that potatoes raised blood glucose more quickly than fruit and that legumes raised blood glucose quite slowly.

This was valuable research, but this method is not generally that useful because it only evaluates one food at a time. This is not how people really eat. Most people eat several foods in a meal, and some are high in carbohydrate while others are high in protein or fat. In addition, a number of other factors affect how quickly foods raise blood glucose, such as:

- How much blood glucose–lowering medication you take

- The time of your last dose of diabetes medication and the time you eat

- The fiber content of the foods you eat

- The ripeness of the fruit or vegetable you eat

- Whether the food is cooked or raw

- How quickly or slowly you eat

- The level of blood glucose (rises faster when blood glucose is low)

Although some health care practitioners and people with diabetes use the glycemic index for meal planning, the ADA has not endorsed it. That's because of the many other factors that affect the rise in blood glucose levels. Besides, if people with diabetes only eat foods that cause a low glycemic rise, they limit their food choices and risk losing variety in their meals. Eating a variety of foods is the number one guideline for people who want to be healthy.

That said, in a sense, you will develop your own personal glycemic index as you progress with carb counting. As you keep records of the foods you eat, their affect on your blood glucose levels, the medication you take, the exercise you do, the stress in your day, and the times that all this happens, you will find foods that cause your blood glucose levels to rise more or less than you expect. It's great to identify these foods for yourself. Then with this information, you can decide whether to eat a food or to eat a smaller serving. Or you might decide (if you are able) to take more diabetes medication to decrease the rise in your blood glucose from particular foods. However, don't be quick to jump to conclusions.

Try the food several times and make sure your blood glucose isn't rising quickly or so high because the serving is larger than previously or other foods you ate at the same time affected your blood glucose, too. See chapter 11 to learn more about using your personal experiences with foods.

Tips to Eat Less Sweets

- Choose a few favorite desserts and decide how often to eat them.

- Satisfy your sweet tooth with a bite or two of your favorite sweet instead of the whole thing.

- If you have a difficult time limiting portions or how often you eat sweets, it is best not to bring large portions of sweets into the house. You might only order dessert at restaurants or just purchase a small quantity at a time.

- Split a dessert with a dining companion in a restaurant. Ask for several forks or spoons.

- Take advantage of smaller portions—kiddie, small, or regular—at ice cream shops or in the supermarket.

- Check your blood glucose from time to time two hours after you eat a sweet to see how high it makes your blood glucose rise.

Easy Ways to Eat Less Sugars

- Trade regular soda for diet soda, or even better, water.

- When you order or buy iced tea, make sure it is unsweetened or sweetened with a low-calorie sweetener.

- When you buy fruit drinks or flavored seltzers, read the Nutrition Facts. Make sure the calories, carbohydrate, and sugars are near zero. You can substitute fruit drink for fruit juice, but it's better to drink water and eat pieces of fruit.

- Trade canned fruit packed in heavy syrup for fruit packed in its own juice or light syrup.

- Use low-calorie sweeteners instead of sugar.

- Use low- or no-sugar jelly or jam instead of regular.

2

What's Carb Counting?

A Bit of History

For years, counting carbohydrate was the method of choice in the United Kingdom. Then in the early 1990s, Carb Counting received a lot of attention in the Diabetes Control and Complications Trial (DCCT). This was the long-term study of people with type 1 diabetes that showed good control of blood glucose reduces diabetes complications, such as eye, kidney, and nerve disease. Carb Counting was one of the meal-planning approaches used in the DCCT.

Interest in Carb Counting also grew when the American Diabetes Association (ADA) used the science supporting Carb Counting to make their 1994 Nutrition Recommendations. In these recommendations, the ADA stressed that the bottom line for blood glucose control is to focus on **the total amount of carbohydrate you eat—not the source of the carbohydrate.** As far as your blood glucose level is concerned, generally speaking, a carbohydrate is a carbohydrate is a carbohydrate. Today many health professionals are teaching people with diabetes how to use Carb Counting. This method gives you flexibility in food choices and can help you improve your blood glucose control.

Carb Counting does not dictate that you should eat a certain percent of your calories as carbohydrate. It is simply a method by which to plan and eat balanced meals and control your blood glucose level. If you and your health care providers believe you will be able to more successfully achieve your diabetes and nutrition goals by eating less carbohydrate (about 40% of calories), then that's fine. Conversely, if you are a vegetarian and eat mainly carbohydrates, then you might achieve your goals with nearly 60% of your calories as carbohydrate. What's most important is that you find a plan that you can use each day that works for you long term. Learn more about how much carb to eat in Table 2-3 on pages 28–29.

Carb Counting: From Basic to Advanced

Carb Counting goes from Basic to Advanced, and you can stop anywhere along the way. Basic Carb Counting is easier to follow and no matter how far you go in your Carb Counting education it is the place you need to start. For starters, to put Carb Counting into practice, you learn how to count the amount of carbohydrate in different foods. Then you learn how much carbohydrate you need to eat at meals and snacks. The focus of Basic Carb Counting is to eat about the same amount of carbohydrate at the same times each day to keep your blood glucose levels in your target ranges. Below, meet Joe. He's using Basic Carb Counting to get his blood glucose levels under control.

Meet Joe   Joe recently found out he had diabetes when he went to see his doctor about being sluggish and thirsty. He thought he might have diabetes because several of his family members do. Joe works hard as an airplane mechanic at the local airport. His blood glucose levels were in the 250 mg/dl range when he was diagnosed. His A1C was 10.5%. Joe is 56 years old and about 30 pounds overweight. He has put on about 5 pounds a year for the last fifteen years. Joe also has high blood pressure, which he controls with medication. His doctor put him on a diabetes medication to help lower his blood glucose. At the same time, the doctor prescribed attendance at a diabetes education program offered at the community hospital. Joe and his wife went to the group program and also had an individual session with the dietitian.

The dietitian spent a lot of time talking to Joe about his eating habits and wanted to know which ones he was willing to change. Joe said that he probably needs to eat at regular times during the day and eat less food for dinner and during the evening. He thought he could give up some of his sweets as long as he was able to still have a little each week. The dietitian thought Joe would do well with Basic Carbohydrate Counting, but he and his wife didn't know much about nutrition. In the first session, the dietitian taught them:

1. The effect of carbohydrate on blood glucose
2. What foods contain carbohydrate
3. The amount of food that is considered "one serving of carbohydrate"
4. How much carbohydrate Joe should eat for breakfast, lunch, dinner, and his nighttime snack

The dietitian also gave Joe some sample meals and showed him how to find the amount of total carbohydrate on the Nutrition Facts panels on foods. She suggested that he check his blood glucose two times a day at different times, including before and after meals, to see the effect of carbohydrate on his blood glucose levels.

The meal plan Joe and his dietitian developed was as follows:

Breakfast:	75 g carb (5 carb servings*)
Lunch:	75 g carb (5 carb servings)
Dinner:	90 g carb (6 carb servings)
Snack:	30 g carb (2 carb servings)

*1 carb serving is equivalent to around 15 g of carbohydrate.

SAMPLE 1-DAY MEAL PLAN FOR JOE

Breakfast: 2 slices whole-wheat toast with peanut butter
(2 carb servings/30 g carb)
1 whole large banana
(2 carb servings/30 g carb)
1/2 cup orange juice (1 carb serving/15 g carb)

Lunch: (Fast food restaurant)
1 hamburger (2 carb servings/30 g carb)
1 small French fries (2 carb servings/30 g carb)
1 8-oz carton low-fat milk
(1 carb serving/15 g carb)
1 small peach or pear (which he brings with
him) (1 carb serving/15 g carb)

Dinner: Salad—1/2 cup cooked green or yellow
vegetable
2 cups pasta (6 carb servings/90 g carb)
1/2 cup tomato and meat sauce
(1 carb serving/15 g carb)
1 dinner roll (1 carb serving/15 g carb)

Snack: 1 cup fat-free milk (1 carb serving/12 g carb)
2 small cookies (1 carb serving/15 g carb)

Joe scheduled another appointment in one month. He was quite pleased with himself on his return. He had lost 2 pounds and, most importantly, his blood glucose levels had dropped into the mid-100s when fasting and before meals, and they were 180–200 mg/dl two hours after eating. But he told the dietitian that he was hungry, particularly in the evenings. In the past, this had been his munching time. They discussed whether Joe felt he needed more food or whether he was just hungry because he was used to eating then. They reworked his carb servings to give Joe more food at lunch and dinner and less at breakfast. The dietitian also suggested some evening snacks that might be more satisfying.

At the dietitian's suggestion, Joe had brought in some food labels from the foods he regularly ate. They talked about how Joe could fit these foods into his carbohydrate count. The dietitian told Joe that he could burn calories and lower his blood glucose if he took a walk in the evening several nights a week. This would also help distract him from thinking too much about food. He said he was willing to take a walk three nights a week. They set up another appointment for a month later. At that time they will continue to monitor how his carbohydrate counting plan is working for Joe and his diabetes. They will also determine what else he needs to learn and what support he needs.

In this scenario, Basic Carb Counting fit Joe's needs and it still does. He finds it easy to follow, and he doesn't want to fuss with too many calculations. His blood glucose is coming into a good range using this approach and that is what is key.

Advanced Carb Counting

Advanced Carb Counting is more complex and is mainly for people who take rapid-acting insulin at meal times along with a daily longer-acting insulin or for people who are on an insulin pump. To do Advanced Carb Counting, you need to learn to adjust the dosage of mealtime insulin you take based on your blood glucose level before the meal and the amount of carbohydrate you plan to eat. You also need to learn and be willing to accurately count the grams of carbohydrate in the food you eat. You also will need to work out your insulin-to-carbohydrate ratio (sometimes called an I:Carb ratio) with your health care provider. This ratio tells you how much rapid-acting insulin you need to take "to cover" the amount of carbohydrate you eat, so you can keep your blood glucose levels in your target range—not too high and not too low. For example, you might learn you need 1 unit of rapid-acting insulin to cover the blood glucose rise from 15 grams (g) of carbohydrate and that 15 g of carbohydrate usually raises your blood glucose about 50 mg/dl. Keep in mind that no two people are alike. These factors need to be individualized for each person based on his or her insulin needs.

Though they have their differences, Basic and Advanced Carbohydrate Counting are not two different meal-planning approaches. They are one approach that can progress over time based on the way you manage your diabetes, your desire for flexibility, and your need to adjust your insulin and food. You decide how far you want to advance. Perhaps, like Joe, you master Basic Carbohydrate Counting and that helps you control your blood glucose levels. Then you reach a point several (or many) years later when you find that to keep your blood glucose in control you need to start taking insulin, which is not uncommon. In fact, about 50–60% of people with type 2 do move on to taking insulin as their diabetes progresses. You may have difficulty controlling your blood glucose levels on insulin, and wonder whether you can achieve better diabetes control if you learn to more precisely adjust the amount of insulin you take at each meal.

Two Ways to Count

As you saw in Joe's meal plan, there are two ways to count carbohydrates—counting *grams* of carbohydrate or counting carbohydrate *servings*. If you learn to count grams of carbohydrate, you add up the number of grams of carbohydrate in each food you eat. Counting the grams of carbohydrate is more precise and is the method you should use if you do Advanced Carb Counting.

No matter which way you count carbs, you'll find it helps to learn some shortcuts, such as the amount of carbohydrate in common foods. For example, 1/2 cup of mashed potatoes, 1 ounce (oz) of dry cereal, and one slice of bread all have 15 g of carbohydrate. If you have 1 cup of mashed potatoes, you need to add 15 g + 15 g for your serving of 30 g of carbohydrate. (See Table 1-1 in chapter 1.) For a more detailed list you have Appendix 1, which is a list of about 500 commonly eaten foods in the U.S. with the exact number of grams per reasonable serving. Other resources for carb counts of foods are the Nutrition Facts panel on food labels and books and web sites with nutrient data. Appendix 2 provides a list of these resources.

Remember the Number 15

The number 15 can help you get a rough estimate of carb counts in foods and make good use of the information on the Nutrition Facts panel. That's because it is the number of grams of carbohydrate in one reasonable serving of several of the carbohydrate-containing food groups—starches, fruit, and milk and yogurt (Table 2-1). However, not all servings contain exactly 15 g of carbohydrate—not in the real world, at least. So, you will find that the number of grams of carbohydrate will vary from serving to serving, from food to food. To help you decide how many carbs or carb servings there are in a portion, use Table 2-2.

HOW MUCH CARBOHYDRATE SHOULD I EAT?

There is no set amount of carbohydrate that is right for everyone. The amount of carbohydrate you need to eat at your meals and snacks should be based on several factors:

T A B L E 2 - 1 Single Servings of Carbohydrate*			
Food group	1 serving	2 servings	3 servings
Starches	15 g	30 g	45 g
Fruit	15 g	30 g	45 g
Milk and yogurt	12 g	24 g	36 g

* Based on servings from *Exchange Lists for Meal Planning*, ADA and The American Dietetic Association, 2003.

TABLE 2-2 Carbohydrate Servings and Grams of Carbohydrate

Carbohydrate choices	Grams of carbohydrate	Grams of carbohydrate per carbohydrate serving
1/2	6–7	6–7
1	15	8–22
2	30	23–37
3	45	38–52
4	60	53–65
5	75	68–82
6	90	83–95

- Your height and weight
- Your usual food habits and daily schedule
- The foods you like to eat
- The amount of physical activity you do
- Your health status and diabetes goals
- The diabetes medications you take and the times that you take them
- Your blood glucose monitoring results
- The results of your blood lipid tests

There are general guidelines about how to choose a certain amount of carbohydrate to eat based on whether you are male or female, small or large, and want to lose weight or not. Table 2-3 can help you design a healthy eating plan. Once you identify which calorie level and nutrient breakdown is best for you, divide the servings into meals and snacks. As a starting point, most women need about

WHAT ARE GRAMS OF CARBOHYDRATE?

Nutrition Facts
Serving Size 1 cup (58g)
Servings Per Container about 8

Amount Per Serving	Multi-Bran Chex	with 1/2 cup skim milk
Calories	200	240
Calories from Fat	15	15
	% Daily Value**	
Total Fat 1.5g*	**2%**	**3%**
Saturated Fat 0g	**0%**	**0%**
Polyunsaturated Fat 0.5g		
Monounsaturated Fat 0g		
Cholesterol 0mg	**0%**	**1%**
Sodium 380mg	**16%**	**19%**
Potassium 220mg	**6%**	**12%**
Total Carbohydrate 49g	**16%**	**18%**
Dietary Fiber 8g	**30%**	**30%**
Sugars 12g		
Other Carbohydrate 29g		
Protein 4g		

Don't confuse gram weight on the serving size of a Nutrition Facts panel with carbohydrate grams.

Answer these True/False questions to check your knowledge of grams.

A gram is a unit of weight in the metric system. **True.**

Carbohydrate is counted in grams (g). **True.**

When you weigh something that is 1 ounce (oz), the metric conversion is 30 g. **True.**

You can weigh a food that contains carbohydrate and know the grams of carbohydrate in that food. **False.**

The number of grams of carbohydrate, protein, and fat in a food is not the same as the weight of the food itself. For example, a medium (4 oz) apple may weigh 120 g (since there are 30 g in an ounce), but the amount of carbohydrate in it is about 15 g. A medium (6 oz) potato weighs 180 g (30 g × 6 oz), but the amount of carbohydrate in it is about 30 g.

TABLE 2 - 3 How Much Carbohydrate Should You Eat?

Calorie Range*	Women who desire weight loss 1200–1400 Calories		Women, older and smaller 1400–1600 Calories		Women (moderate to large size), older men, and men (small to moderate) who desire weight loss 1600–1900 Calories		Children, teen girls, active larger women, men (small to moderate) 1900–2300 Calories		Teen boys, active men (moderate to large) 2300–2800 Calories	
	40–45%**	45–50%**	40–45%	45–50%	40–45%	45–50%	40–45%	45–50%	40–45%	45–50%
Carb (g)***	130	160	150	180	180	210	215	260	260	300
Carb servings/day (Each = 15 g of carb)***	8	10	9	11	11	13	13	16	16	19
Servings per day of:										
Grains, beans and starchy vegetables	4	5	5	6	6	8	8	10	10	12
Fruits	2	3	2	3	3	3	3	4	4	5
Milk***	2	2	2	2	2	2	2	2	2	2
Vegetables (non-starchy)	3	3	4	4	4	4	5	5	5	5

Meats*****	6 oz	5 oz	7 oz	6 oz	8 oz	7	9 oz	8 oz	10 oz	9 oz
Fats	35–40%**	30–35%**	35–40%	30–35%	35–40%	30–35%	35–40%	30–35%	35–40%	30–35%
Meat/Fat g (total = meats + fats)	50	45	65	55	75	60	90	75	110	90
Fat servings (5 g fat each)******	7	6	9	7	10	8	13	10	16	13

* The groups of people for who these calorie ranges are appropriate are generalizations. To learn how many calories you need, as well as how much of the other nutrients you need to accomplish your diabetes and nutrition goals, work with a dietitian specialized in diabetes.

** For each calorie level you find two variations for the nutrient breakdown. One suggests you get about 40-–45% of calories from carbohydrate and 35–40% of calories from fat. This is on the lower side of carbohydrate and the higher side for fat, but some people with type 2 diabetes and lipid problems may find this helpful. Ensure that as much of your fat as possible comes from monounsaturated fat sources (see Appendix 1). The other variation is 45–50% of calories from carbohydrate and 30–35% of calories from fat.

*** The total grams of carbohydrate and servings of carbohydrate are from grains, beans, starchy vegetables, fruits, and milk. Non-starchy vegetables aren't counted in the carbohydrate total.

**** Based on fat-free milk (12 g of carb and 8 g of protein per 8 oz). Children between 9 and 18 years old need 1300 mg of calcium per day. They should get at least 3 servings of milk per day. Adults from 19–50 need 1000 mg of calcium per day. This can be met with 2 servings of milk a day plus another serving of a high calcium food. Women over 51 need 1200 mg of calcium per day. If you don't drink milk because you dislike it or are lactose intolerant, you need to find another source of calcium. To get an equivalent amount of carbohydrate add another 24 g from either grains, beans or starchy vegetables or fruit.

***** Calculated based on lean meat figures (7 g of protein and 3 g of fat per ounce). Use more or less grams or servings of fat based on the type of meats you tend to eat. See Appendix 1.

****** The servings of fat figure that each serving provides 5 g of fat. See Appendix 1.

3–4 carbohydrate servings (45–60 g) and most men need about 4–5 carbohydrate servings (60–75 g) at each meal. You may need less if you want to lose weight. If you take insulin at each meal, you can learn to adjust the dose to "match" your carbohydrate intake. For people using Basic Carb Counting, it is important to keep the amount of carbohydrate you eat at meals and snacks about the same from meal to meal and day to day. This will help you control your blood glucose.

Consider the amount of carbohydrate suggested in Table 2-3 as a starting point. Find a dietitian who specializes in diabetes care to work with you to determine the amount of carbohydrate that best fits your needs and to help you master carbohydrate counting. (See page 205 to learn how to find a dietitian.)

3

Are You Ready to Begin Basic Carb Counting?

It's Time to Assess Yourself

Are you ready to find out the carb content of the foods you eat, weigh and measure your servings of foods, count the carbs, check your blood glucose at least two times a day, and record the numbers? It sounds like a lot, but it will be important for you to do these things when you start Carb Counting. As time goes on and Carb Counting becomes more natural and you can eyeball certain portions, this process won't seem as rigorous. However, it will be important for you to always pay careful attention to the amounts of food you eat and your blood glucose numbers. Carb Counting is not hard, but it does take a commitment from you.

ARE YOU READY TO:

1. Find a meal-planning approach that fits your lifestyle and desire for more flexibility?

☐ yes   ☐ no

You may have tried a variety of meal-planning approaches in the past—the food exchange system, the food guide pyramid, or counting calories—and believe you need a meal-planning approach that offers more flexibility. Or maybe you are new to diabetes and your health care provider recommended Carb Counting because it seems to fit your lifestyle.

2. Find a meal-planning approach that helps you achieve better control of your blood glucose levels?

☐ yes   ☐ no

Who doesn't want this? The more carbohydrate you eat, the higher your blood glucose level is going to go. If you know where it's going, you can add exercise or adjust your medication to bring it back down. It makes sense, then, that if you eat the same amount of carbohydrate at the same meals from day to day, you can control your blood glucose better.

3. Learn more about foods and how much carbohydrate is in them?

☐ yes   ☐ no

Foods contain varying amounts of carbohydrate. You'll learn approximate amounts of carbohydrate contained in foods. You'll also discover where to find and how to estimate the carb count of an endless list of foods.

4. Pay more attention to what you eat and the amount you eat?

☐ yes   ☐ no

You will be able to eat the foods you enjoy in reasonable amounts. You'll learn skills and strategies to estimate portions of foods whether you eat at home or out.

5. Keep food records that detail the types of foods, the amount, when you eat, and how much carb is in each food, meal, or snack?

☐ yes   ☐ no

Keeping a record will provide you with a profile of your food choices and the amounts of foods you eat. It will also help you build your own database of carb counts so you don't have to keep looking them up.

6. Check blood glucose levels at least two times a day and record the results?

☐ yes   ☐ no

Many things can affect your blood glucose level. If you haven't been checking it, you'll need to check it either before or two hours after the start of your meals for a couple of weeks. This information, along with the food information you record, gives you a feel for the effect of the different carbs you eat on your blood glucose levels.

7. Have the tools to weigh and measure servings—and actually use them?

☐ yes   ☐ no

You need to measure your servings in order to get skilled at "guess-timating" the amounts you eat (when you don't have a scale handy), because this is how you count the carbs in the serving. For example, a slice of bread is 1 serving of carbohydrate or 15 grams (g) of carbohydrate. But this is based on a 1-ounce (oz) piece of bread from a commercial loaf of bread that you might buy at the grocery store. A thicker, heavier slice of bread weighing 3 oz could be 3 carb servings or 45 g of carbohydrate.

Do you own or are you willing to purchase the following tools for carbohydrate counting?

Scale to weigh foods	☐	yes	☐	no
Measuring cups	☐	yes	☐	no
Measuring spoons	☐	yes	☐	no

When you use Carb Counting, you need to practice, practice, and practice some more to get skilled at eating the correct portions.

And once you are skilled at it, you still need to use the measuring tools every month or so to check that your servings haven't grown over time.

8. Read the Nutrition Facts label on packaged foods to find the Total Carbohydrate content?

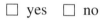

☐ yes   ☐ no

You'll learn that the Nutrition Facts on foods are a huge asset to Carb Counters. When you use packaged foods you'll have the information right in front of you. No need to research the carb counts. Being familiar with the carb counts from Nutrition Facts panels helps you better estimate carb counts of foods that don't have Nutrition Facts, such as unpackaged foods or restaurant foods.

9. Spend time to learn how much carbohydrate you need to eat to keep your blood glucose levels in control?

☐ yes   ☐ no

Your food and blood glucose records help you see the effect of carbohydrate foods on your blood glucose. This helps you and your health care provider decide how much carbohydrate to eat, how much medication to take, and how much physical activity you need to keep your blood glucose levels within the target range you want. It also helps both of you know when you need to make adjustments.

4

How Many Meals and Snacks to Eat?

For many years the preferred meal plan for people with diabetes was three square meals plus three snacks a day. This advice is no longer true. Today, with more medication options and medications that don't cause blood glucose to go too low, you don't necessarily need to eat between-meal snacks. However, you may want to. Need versus want—that's a big difference! Talk with your health care provider to figure out how many meals and snacks (if any) are the right number for you to achieve the best control of your blood glucose. This should be based on your habits and schedule, how you manage your diabetes, and your need for flexibility.

A Bit of History

Until 1994 the only category of diabetes pills available for people with type 2 diabetes were sulfonylureas and a few types of insulin. Neither allowed much flexibility to vary amounts of food, plus they could cause blood glucose to fall too low (hypoglycemia). To avoid hypoglycemia, people with diabetes on these medications were encouraged to eat three meals and two to three snacks each day.

A NEW DAY HAS DAWNED

Today a variety of insulins and oral medications are available that work at different times and in different ways. By mixing and matching new medications, you and your health care providers have many more combinations with which to control your blood glucose. Several of the new oral diabetes medications don't even cause hypoglycemia, and a couple of others closely match the quick rise in blood glucose from food and then quickly leave the body (Table 4-1). All of these options allow you and your health care providers to find the medication regimen that most closely matches your diabetes and lifestyle needs. You don't have to eat a set number of meals or snacks at all. What you should be able to do is base the decisions about snacks and the size of breakfast,

TABLE 4-1 Diabetes Medications and Hypoglycemia	
Diabetes medications that can cause hypoglycemia	Diabetes medications that do not cause hypoglycemia
Sulfonylureas: Amaryl, Glucotrol, Glucotrol XL, DiaBeta, Glynase, Micronase, Orinase, Tolinase, Diabinese, Dymelor	**Metformin:** Glucophage, Glucophage XR
Glucovance (Glucovance is a combination of metformin and glyburide, a sulfonylurea. The glyburide portion can cause hypoglycemia.)	**Alpha-glucosidase inhibitors:** Precose and Glyset
	Glitazones: Avandia and Actos
Metaglip (Metaglip is a combination of metformin and glipizide, a sulfonylurea. The glipizide portion can cause hypoglycemia.)	**Avandamet** (Avandamet is a combination of Avandia and metformin, neither of which cause hypoglycemia.)
Meglitinides: Repaglinide (Prandin)	
D-phenylalanine: Nateglinide (Starlix)	
Insulin	

TWO RAPID-ACTING MEDS

There are two categories of medications that can cause hypoglycemia. However, it is unlikely this will happen because they act quickly. In the category of oral medications, the two available pills are repaglinide (Prandin) and nateglinide (Starlix). Prandin is taken just before you eat. It helps the pancreas quickly produce insulin to help lower the blood glucose rise that occurs from the carbohydrate you eat. It works quickly and leaves the body quickly. As long as the meal is sufficient to match the amount of medication, the risk of hypoglycemia is small.

In the category of insulin, two brands of rapid-acting insulin are available: lispro (Humalog) and aspart (Novolog). The rapid-acting insulin also works in conjunction with the rise in blood glucose from a meal. It starts working within five to fifteen minutes and peaks in forty-five to seventy-five minutes. Both insulins are out of your system within about four hours. Keep in mind that these are general onset, peaks, and durations for these insulins. People may find some individual differences. With their quick action, you don't need to be a slave to snacking to prevent hypoglycemia several hours later.

lunch, and dinner on your blood glucose goals and what fits your lifestyle. Once again, use the feedback from your blood glucose checks to tell you whether you need to adjust your food or your medication, or both. Plus, based on your eating pattern, your health care provider can select the diabetes medications and regimen that work best for you.

How Many Meals and Snacks Do You Eat?

You will most likely achieve the best blood glucose control if you eat about the same amount of carbohydrate at the same meals and snacks from day to day. That's particularly true if you don't adjust the amount of medication you take for the amount of carbohydrate you eat. However, for most people this plan just doesn't mesh with real life. Very few people eat this way today. Here's the more common picture: Eat breakfast—if they eat breakfast—as they're flying out the door or in the car. Lunch is usually a quick meal but larger than breakfast and smaller than dinner. Dinner is typically the largest meal of the day. If the way you eat looks like this, then your health care providers need to take this into account, within reason, when they prescribe types and amounts of diabetes medications.

A word to the wise: Let your health care provider know as much about your eating style and daily schedule as you can. Don't let them prescribe medications for you based on an idealized nine-to-five lifestyle that simply isn't true to your life. Let them know whether you prefer three meals and two snacks or three meals and no snacks. Tell them the times you usually eat meals or snacks. This information is helpful because some diabetes medications have an onset, peak, and duration of action. This "action curve" needs to be in sync with when you eat. Help your health care provider learn enough about you and your lifestyle to set your medication plan around your real eating habits, instead of setting up your medication schedule in a way that forces you to eat to meet the action of the meds.

Even if you are not asked to keep a food diary, you might want to do so anyway. You may not know what your real eating habits are. A record gives information about your food choices and lifestyle that you can discuss with your health care provider. Let your provider know if you often have hypoglycemia, feel hungry, or are gaining weight. These could be signs that your diabetes medication is not matching well with your lifestyle. Also, the records of your blood glucose checks are the best way for you to know whether your blood glucose is under control. Remember, there are a variety of diabetes medications, which allows you to design a diabetes plan that is flexible enough to fit your lifestyle.

Key Questions and Answers about Snacks

TO SNACK OR NOT?

Here are several questions for you to consider when you decide how many meals and snacks are right for you.

1. Would you rather have six small meals or three larger meals a day?
2. Do you enjoy snacks at certain times of the day or do you feel snacks are just a bother?
3. If you like to snack, what time(s) of the day do you want a snack?
4. Do you feel that you need snacks for good nutrition or to better manage your blood glucose?

WHAT FOODS MAKE GOOD SNACKS?

There are plenty of both healthy and not-so-healthy snacks available today. The ideal snack is fresh, convenient to purchase or carry, and easy to eat. A few healthy and convenient snacks are:

- Fruit (fresh, canned, or dried)

- Nuts and seeds

- Yogurt or milk

- Dry cereals

- Popcorn

- Pretzels

Unfortunately, these may not be as readily available as the not-so-healthy snacks that are high in calories, fat, and sodium, such as potato and corn chips, cookies, candy, and ice cream. To eat healthy snacks you need to plan ahead. For example, to avoid the temptation of the vending machine, you might take a small piece or two of fruit with you when you leave the house. The benefit of planning is that you get a snack packed with fiber, vitamins, and minerals. Appendix 1 has carb counts for various foods that you might choose for healthy snacks.

SHOULD YOU HAVE FRUIT OR FRUIT JUICE FOR A SNACK?

The simple answer is yes, because most Americans don't eat enough fruit. Some people with diabetes have been told not to eat fruit or fruit juice as a snack because they can cause a quick rise in blood glucose. But research shows that most sources of carbohydrate raise blood glucose to about the same level in about the same amount of time. Fruit and fruit juice are no exception. In fact, some studies have shown that fruit raises blood glucose more slowly than some other carbohydrates because they contain about 50% fructose. So if you need to eat more fruit to improve your diet and the only way you can fit it in is with snacks, try it. Then a couple of times check your blood glucose two hours later to see how high it rises. If it is too high, then try eating fruit as part of a meal instead.

SHOULD SNACKS CONTAIN CARBOHYDRATE AND PROTEIN?

For years people have been taught that between-meal snacks, and especially bedtime snacks, should contain carbohydrate and protein—crackers and cheese or peanut butter, half of a turkey or roast beef sandwich, or graham crackers and milk. The thought was that protein is a longer-lasting source of energy, and it would keep blood glucose levels up longer to prevent hypoglycemia. Some studies do show that protein helps to reduce the rise in blood glucose after a meal or snack, so you may want to continue these protein-carb snacks if your records show that this is true for you . . . and your stomach and brain agree, especially during the night.

If you don't find that protein in the snack helps you keep your blood glucose in control and that you'd rather eat your protein at meals, talk to your health care providers about adjusting your diabetes plan. See chapter 6 for more.

ARE DIABETES SNACK PRODUCTS BENEFICIAL?

This is debatable. There are pluses and there are minuses. On the plus side, these bars and drinks offer a quick and easy choice that may be healthier than your current snacks because they contain essential vitamins and minerals. A few small studies show that beyond just providing calories and vitamins and minerals, the bars and drinks may slow down and lower the rise of blood glucose a few hours after consumption. This effect is due either to a carbohydrate-based ingredient in several products or to the ratio of nutrients.

Then there are the minuses. These products can be expensive. Also, some of these foods are high in fat and calories. If you eat them regularly, you and your health care provider need to fit them into your eating plan. Don't eat them as extras.

Meet Sue

Sue is 35 years old and has had type 1 diabetes for ten years. She has always had to work hard to control her weight. Sue has been on two injections of insulin a day for many years. She takes an intermediate-acting insulin (NPH) and regular insulin before breakfast and before dinner. She has been encouraged to eat a mid-afternoon and a bedtime snack to keep her blood glucose from dipping too low. She is a traveling salesperson for a large food service company. She does not always get lunch or a mid-afternoon snack on time, causing her to often get shaky and sweaty because of hypoglycemia. She then panics and over-treats the low blood glucoses with high-calorie foods, such as ice cream or chocolate. Sue would prefer not to snack because it is inconvenient in her job and hinders maintaining her weight.

After reading an article about people with type 1 diabetes using a four-shot-a-day combination of a long-acting insulin—glargine, taken once a day—and a rapid-acting insulin used at meals based on blood glucose and carb count, she approached her doctor with the article in hand. She also had a one-week food diary and her blood glucose records.

Sue noted that she is tired of having to snack to keep her blood glucose up, and she pointed to the time constraints of her job and daily schedule. She asked if this type of insulin regimen was for her. Her doctor said, "Let's give it a try." She began taking glargine once a day before bed and a certain amount of rapid-acting insulin at each meal based on her blood glucose level. Her doctor sent her to a dietitian to learn more about Carb Counting. The dietitian helped Sue learn the elements of both Basic and Advanced Carb Counting. They calculated Sue's insulin-to-carbohydrate (I:Carb) ratio, which was 20 grams (g) of carb to 1 unit of rapid-acting insulin. Sue made a second appointment with the dietitian. She came back with records that showed her food intake, grams of carbohydrate, amount of insulin taken, and the results of at least four blood glucose checks a day. The next visit they made some adjustments. Over time and slowly but surely, Sue was better able to control her blood glucose. For her, the best part was not having to bother with snacks between meals and being able to lose a few pounds. Sue did, however, continue to carry some glucose tablets and nonperishable snacks in her car for those times her blood glucose was getting low or for when she just couldn't get a meal.

Low Blood Glucose: What You Need to Know and Do

Keeping your blood glucose levels in control is akin to walking on a balance beam. Think of the beam as the healthy range in which to keep your blood glucose levels, basically 90–180 mg/dl (this includes both before and after meals). It's healthiest not to have your blood glucose go higher than 180 mg/dl after eating. Nor is it safe to have your blood glucose get too low (under 70 mg/dl) too often. However, to stay in your target range as much as possible, you will find that on occasion your blood glucose will go too low. Do note, however, that blood glucose can only get too low if you take insulin or one of the oral diabetes medicines that can cause low blood glucose. (See Table 4-1 for a list of medications that do and don't make blood glucose too low.)

It is worth noting that studies in people with type 2 diabetes show that even if they take a diabetes medication that can cause low blood glucose, severe hypoglycemia is rare. This is also true for people with type 2 diabetes who take insulin. It is not, however, true for people with type 1 diabetes who take insulin. They can more easily develop severe hypoglycemia.

WHAT CAUSES HYPOGLYCEMIA?

- Too much of a diabetes medicine that can cause hypo-glycemia (see Table 4-1)

- Not enough carb and/or total amount of food eaten at a meal or snack

- A delayed or missed meal or snack

- Increased physical activity (an amount that is unusual for you) without a reduction in the amount of insulin or medication or with no extra carb

WHAT ARE THE SYMPTOMS OF HYPOGLYCEMIA?

Common symptoms of low blood glucose are:

- Shakiness

- Sweating

- Feeling disoriented or dizzy

- Blurred vision

- Mood changes, irritability

- Headache

You may have one, several, or none of these symptoms. It's helpful if you are familiar with your own symptoms of low blood glucose. Share these with your family, friends, and coworkers so they can recognize it, too. When your blood glucose goes too low your thinking and coordination may be impaired. If your blood glucose goes even lower, you can lose consciousness. It's important that family, friends, and coworkers know that you have diabetes and may experience hypoglycemia. You need to explain what they should do for you if you can't help yourself. This may be anything from getting you a few glucose tablets that are in your desk drawer or nightstand to calling 911 for emergency help.

WHAT CAN YOU DO TO PREVENT HYPOGLYCEMIA?

To limit hypoglycemia, it's important to eat your target amount of carb at regularly spaced meals. Depending on whether or not you have greater than five hours between your meals and the diabetes medicines you take, you may need to eat a snack between meals. Also, if you take diabetes medications, it's important to take the correct dose at the proper time. If you get more physical activity than you are used to, it will be important to eat more carbs. Check your blood glucose before the activity. If your blood glucose level is 100 mg/dl or less, consider eating some carb before you exercise. This is particularly important if you will do a good bit of activity. Then try to remember to check your blood glucose after the activity to determine what it is and if you need more carb. Your blood glucose is likely to decrease over the next few hours because the body is using more glucose. Even when you are consciously trying to prevent hypoglycemia, it can surprise you. Therefore, you need to be ready to deal with it, if it happens.

WHAT DO YOU DO FOR LOW BLOOD GLUCOSE?

An easy way to remember what to do for starters is the "Rule of 15." Treat hypoglycemia with 15 g of carbohydrate (see suggestions below), and wait 15 minutes. Check your blood glucose level and make sure it is on the upswing. If it is still less than 70 mg/dl, then repeat the 15/15.

Examples of 15 g of carbohydrate:

- Three to four glucose tablets (each has 4 g of carb)

- Glucose gel or other preparations of pure glucose

- 4–6 oz of fruit juice (any type)

- 4–6 oz of regular soda (not diet)

- Six small hard candies

The glucose tablets and gels, as well as other pure forms of glucose, are preferred because these will raise blood glucose more quickly. Sources such as fruit juice and regular soda contain some glucose and some fructose. The fructose doesn't raise blood glucose that much. Also, the sources of pure glucose are easy to carry and keep with you at all times.

Always carry some source of glucose with you. You can carry glucose tablets in your purse, pocket, briefcase, backpack, and console of your car and keep them at your bedside. If you feel that your blood glucose level is already slipping too low, treat first and then check your blood glucose level. Do be particularly careful with driving. If you think your blood glucose may be headed down, check it before you start to drive.

HYPOGLYCEMIA UNAWARENESS

Some people who have had type 1 diabetes for five to seven years or who have had many episodes of low blood glucose may develop "hypoglycemia unawareness." This means that they get low blood glucose, but they don't get any symptoms. If this happens to you, protect yourself by doing frequent blood glucose checks and ask your diabetes care provider for training in blood glucose awareness. You don't want to go so low that you pass out. Your family, friends, and coworkers should also be aware of this and know how to use glucagon to bring your blood glucose level back up if you are unconscious. Glucagon is a prescription item and can be obtained with a prescription from your health care provider.

5

Begin Counting

To begin Carb Counting you need to get to know yourself better. That is, you need to get to know your eating habits—what, when, and how much you eat. The best way to accomplish this is to keep records of your current food habits in a food diary. Look at the flow of your average day. Maybe you'll see that you start the day with the same breakfast at the same time, but lunch and dinner are never even close to similar times. Or maybe you'll learn that you follow a pretty tight schedule during the week, but on the weekends your schedule changes dramatically. Or maybe your meal times are different every day.

To be successful with Basic Carbohydrate Counting, you'll need to figure out how much carbohydrate you eat and when—on most days. Eating similar amounts of carb on a fairly regular schedule helps you control your blood glucose levels. Keep detailed, and honest, records. It's the only way you can trust your results and put them to good use to control your blood glucose.

The following seven-step process helps you get a sense of your eating pattern, to figure how much carb you eat, to learn the types of carbs you gravitate toward, and to stack your food records up with your blood glucose records. Take one step at a time and you'll be well on your way with carb counting.

Step 1: Keep Food Records

Begin keeping a food diary by writing down the foods you eat at breakfast, lunch, and dinner. Don't forget to include snacks and nibbles. Yes, crumbs do count! Keep these records for a full week including the weekend. Beyond recording the food, write down the amount you eat. Obviously that's critical information. If it would help to use your measuring cups and spoons to get more accurate quantities, do so. The more accurate you can be, the more helpful your food records will be to you and to your health care provider. Remember, it's not just what you eat, but the all-important "size" of your serving as well. You can design your own food record or use one similar to the record on Table 5-1. The components of your food records should be:

- Day of the week

- Meal time

- Amounts of food

- Carb grams for each food

- Total carb grams for the meal or snack

Step 2: Find the Foods You Ate that Contain Carbohydrate

After you have one week of your food diary completed, go through and circle the foods that contain carbohydrate (Table 5-2 on pages 52–53). Don't forget that dairy foods, fruits, and desserts contain carb and that you might also pick up a few grams from fat-free salad dressing. This helps you learn to identify the foods you typically eat and which ones contain carbohydrates.

Step 3: Figure How Much Carb You Eat

Now, figure how many grams of carbohydrate you eat at each meal. To do this use the list of foods in Appendix 1 or determine carb counts from one or more of the resources listed in Appendix 2. Fill in the grams of carb as we've done in Table 5-3 on pages 54–55. Next, add up the totals for each meal and snack. If you plan to use carb servings rather than carb grams, remember that each carb serving contains 15 grams (g) of carbohydrate.

Step 4: Sit Back and Observe

Ask yourself if you eat the same amount of carbs at your breakfasts, lunches, dinners, and snacks. In the two days of sample records on pages 54–55, the carbs in the breakfasts vary from 75 g to 102 g. And the times at which breakfast is eaten are very different, too. One day breakfast is at 7 A.M. and the next it's at 9 A.M. As you have already learned, varying the amount of carb and the timing of breakfast this much will make it difficult to control blood glucose levels. That's particularly true if you, like most people, take the same amount of diabetes medicine each day. If this is true, you especially need to keep the amount of carbohydrate you eat at meals and snacks fairly consistent to achieve a steady pattern in your blood glucose levels.

Step 5: Get Familiar with the Carb Counts of the Foods You Eat

When it comes to food, most of us are creatures of habit—we eat a similar array of foods day in and day out. Sure, we might eat more similarly on Monday through Friday than we do on the weekend. And once in a while we eat in an ethnic restaurant or we try a new recipe. But generally speaking, week after week, we eat the same foods and meals. That's good news when it comes to

TABLE 5-1   Food Diary

Monday

Breakfast
Time: 7 A.M.

Food	Amount
Blueberry bagel	1 whole
Light cream cheese	2 Tbsp
Strawberries	1 cup sliced

Lunch
Time: 12 noon

Food	Amount
Thin-crust cheese pizza	3 14" slices
Garden salad	1 1/2 cups
Thousand Island dressing	2 Tbsp
Frozen yogurt cone	1 small

Dinner
Time: 6:30 P.M.

Food	Amount
Grilled chicken	5 oz cooked
Barbecue sauce	2 Tbsp
Long-grain rice casserole	1 cup
Corn on the cob	1 large
Margarine	2 Tbsp
Applesauce (no sugar added)	1 cup

Snack
Time: 9 P.M.

Food	Amount
Oatmeal raisin cookie	1 large

TABLE 5-1 Food Diary (continued)

Tuesday

Breakfast
Time: 9 A.M.

Food	Amount
Raisin bran muffin	1
Orange juice	8 oz
Milk, fat-free	8 oz

Lunch
Time: 12:30 P.M.

Food	Amount
Chicken pot pie	8 oz
Dinner roll	1
Apple, medium	6 oz

Dinner
Time: 7:45 P.M.

Food	Amount
Spaghetti	2 cups
Meat sauce	3/4 cup
Parmesan cheese	2 Tbsp
Green salad	1 cup
Fat-free French dressing	2 Tbsp

Snack
Time: 10:30 P.M.

Food	Amount
Light ice cream	1 cup
Blueberries	1/2 cup

TABLE 5-2 Food Diary

Monday

Breakfast
Time: 7 A.M.

Food	*Amount*
Blueberry bagel	1 whole
Light cream cheese	2 Tbsp
Strawberries	1 cup sliced

Lunch
Time: 12 noon

Food	*Amount*
Thin-crust cheese pizza	3 14" slices
Garden salad	1 1/2 cups
Thousand Island dressing	2 Tbsp
Frozen yogurt cone	1 small

Dinner
Time: 6:30 P.M.

Food	*Amount*
Grilled chicken	5 oz cooked
Barbecue sauce	2 Tbsp
Long-grain rice casserole	1 cup
Corn on the cob	1 large
Margarine	2 Tbsp
Applesauce (no sugar added)	1 cup

Snack
Time: 9 P.M.

Food	*Amount*
Oatmeal raisin cookie	1 large

TABLE 5-2 Food Diary (continued)

Tuesday

Breakfast
Time: 9 A.M.

Food	Amount
Raisin bran muffin	1
Orange juice	8 oz
Milk, fat-free	8 oz

Lunch
Time: 12:30 P.M.

Food	Amount
Chicken pot pie	8 oz
Dinner roll	1
Apple, medium	6 oz

Dinner
Time: 7:45 P.M.

Food	Amount
Spaghetti	2 cups
Meat sauce	3/4 cup
Parmesan cheese	2 Tbsp
Green salad	1 cup
Fat-free French dressing	2 Tbsp

Snack
Time: 10:30 P.M.

Food	Amount
Light ice cream	1 cup
Blueberries	1/2 cup

TABLE 5-3 Food Diary

Monday

Breakfast
Time: 7 A.M.

Food	Amount	Carb grams
Blueberry bagel	1 whole	61
Light cream cheese	2 Tbsp	2
Strawberries	1 cup sliced	12
		Total carb: 75

Lunch
Time: 12 noon

Food	Amount	Carb grams
Thin-crust cheese pizza	3 14" slices	66
Garden salad	1 1/2 cups	0
Thousand Island dressing	2 Tbsp	3
Frozen yogurt cone	1 small	23
		Total carb: 92

Dinner
Time: 6:30 P.M.

Food	Amount	Carb grams
Grilled chicken	5 oz cooked	0
Barbecue sauce	2 Tbsp	4
Long-grain rice casserole	1 cup	41
Corn on the cob	1 large	32
Margarine	2 Tbsp	0
Applesauce (no sugar added)	1 cup	30
		Total carb: 107

Snack
Time: 9 P.M.

Food	Amount	Carb grams
Oatmeal raisin cookie	1 large	34
		Total carb: 34

TABLE 5-3 Food Diary (continued)

Tuesday

Breakfast
Time: 9 A.M.

Food	Amount	Carb grams
Raisin bran muffin	1	60
Orange juice	8 oz	30
Milk, fat-free	8 oz	12
		Total carb: 102

Lunch
Time: 12:30 P.M.

Food	Amount	Carb grams
Chicken pot pie	8 oz	35
Dinner roll	1	16
Apple, medium	6 oz	20
		Total carb: 71

Dinner
Time: 7:45 P.M.

Food	Amount	Carb grams
Spaghetti	2 cups	90
Meat sauce	3/4 cup	16
Parmesan cheese	2 Tbsp	0
Green salad	1 cup	0
Fat-free French dressing	2 Tbsp	12
		Total carb: 118

Snack
Time: 10:30 P.M.

Food	Amount	Carb grams
Light ice cream	1 cup	40
Blueberries	1/2 cup	10
		Total carb: 50

Carb Counting because this fact makes it easier to build your own personal "database" of carb counts.

As you start to build your personal database, think about what format for keeping records is best for you. Will it be best to keep your database in a small notebook that you carry with you or a personal digital assistant (PDA)? Or is it better for you to keep it as a continually growing spread sheet on your computer, with the type of information in Table 5-4: the food, the amount you eat in a serving, and the carb count in grams? You be the judge of what works best for you.

Start to build your database by making a list of the foods you regularly eat. Then start to determine the carb counts of the servings of foods. Where possible use the Total Carbohydrate count from Nutrition Facts panels from food packages. If the size of the serving you eat is bigger or smaller, do the math to determine the carb count for the amount you eat. When you don't have a Nutrition Facts label for foods you eat, such as a piece of fruit, a potato, or other fresh foods, look up carb counts in one of many available resources. Today there are many books, computer programs, and online searchable food databases. Learn about the variety of these resources in Appendix 2.

Start with the carb counts in Appendix 1. This list includes the exact carb counts for 500 commonly eaten foods in the U.S. Next move on to one or more of the extensive resources listed in Appendix 2. A terrific and relatively new resource is the online searchable nutrient database available from the U.S. Department of Agriculture (USDA). It contains the nutrition information for about 6,000 basic and commonly eaten foods. This database can also be downloaded and printed out. However, it's probably more logical to search the database for the carb counts of the foods you regularly eat. It's interesting to note that this is the database that provides the core information for many of the books with nutrition information. The web site address for the USDA database is: *www.nal.usda.gov/fnic/foodcomp.* More detail about how to access it is in Appendix 2.

CARB COUNTS: FROM FOODS TO MEALS

After you have looked up the carb counts of the individual foods you regularly eat, next count up the total grams of carbohydrate in the entire meals you regularly eat. Keep a record of these as well. Again, we are creatures of habit, not only in the foods we choose to eat, but in the way we combine these foods for meals and the amount of food we eat. This is good news for you, too.

TABLE 5-4 Sample Personal Database Record–Common Meals and Snacks I Eat		
Meal	Serving (amount I eat)	Grams of carbohydrate*
Breakfast 1: (at home)		
Honey Nut Cheerios	1 cup	24
All Bran with extra Fiber	1/2 cup	23
Milk–fat-free	1 cup	12
Blueberries	1/2 cup	10
Total		**69**
Breakfast 2: (in the car)		
Whole-wheat toast (for egg sandwich)	2 slices	26
Egg (fried)	1 large	0
Cheddar cheese–reduced-fat	1 oz	0
Banana	1 medium (4 oz)	27
Total		**53**
Lunch 1:		
Whole-wheat bread	2 slices	26
Smoked turkey–sliced	2 oz	0
Swiss cheese–part-skim	1 oz	1
Baby carrots	7–10	8
Grape tomatoes	5–8	3
Apple–Granny Smith	1 large (7 oz)	29
Total		**66**

*Nutrition Information obtained from *www.nal.usda.gov/fnic/foodcomp* (the USDA searchable database. For more information about this database see Appendix 2) and Nutrition Facts labels.

This means that it would save you time in the long run to spend a few minutes to develop a database of the carb counts of the common meals you eat. It is likely that you choose one of two or three breakfasts or lunches day after day—at least Monday through Friday. As you figure the carb counts of these meals, take a few extra minutes to weigh and measure the foods, rather than just estimating. This will help you get more exact carb counts. The more exact you can be, the better you can control your blood glucose. Do this as you prepare these meals over a few weeks' time.

Your goal in building your databases is to minimize the time—in the long run—you need to spend counting and recounting carbs in your meals.

Step 6: How Much Carb Should You Eat?

Now you have a picture of how much carbohydrate you eat at your meals and snacks. Look at the chart on pages 28–29 (Table 2-3) to determine the grams of carb or carb servings you need based on your age, sex, and level of activity. Compare your records to this chart and ask yourself: are you eating too much, too little, or just the right amount of carb for you? At this point you might want to consult with your health care provider or set up a visit with a dietitian with expertise in Carb Counting to help you design a Carb Counting plan.

Step 7: Match Up What You Eat with Blood Glucose Records

The next step is to match your food records with your blood glucose records. Learning how your meals and certain foods affect your blood glucose will help you and your health care provider fine-tune your diabetes management plan. Unfortunately, most of the blood glucose records that come with your glucose meter or other diabetes supplies don't provide much room for you to record what you eat and how much carb you eat. We encourage you to try the record form in Appendix 3. You might want to change the form here and there to fit your needs. Table 5-5 is a sample form.

A recording form should provide room to record:

- The timing of your meals and snacks

- The type and dose of your diabetes medications

- The food you eat, including the amount and the grams of carb or carb servings

- The results of your blood glucose checks with a note of the time of the check

- An "other" column to record the type and amount of your physical activity

- Your daily schedule

- Emotions or stressful situations

- Other reasons why your blood glucose results might have been different than expected

You can also record information about activity, emotions, and general observations under a "notes" section.

Recording More Details

DIABETES MEDICATIONS

Some people with diabetes take no medication, some people take one or more pills, and some people take insulin or a combination of pills and insulin. It is this ever-expanding variety of medications that provides the many options with which to control blood glucose. Know the type of diabetes medication(s) you take. Know when to take each one, understand how it works to help control blood glucose, and understand how the medication works in conjunction with the carb you eat to control your blood glucose. Record type, dose, and timing of each medication. Having this information recorded helps you interpret your blood glucose results.

TABLE 5-5 Carbohydrate Counting and Blood Glucose Results Record

Day/Date: *Tuesday, June 3* (Insulin-to-Carb Ratio = 1 unit to 12 g of carb)

Time/ meal	Diabetes medicines		Food		Carb grams
	Type	Amount	Type	Amount	
6:45 A.M./	Huma-log	8u			
7 A.M./b'fast			Shredded Wheat 'n Bran with	1/2 cup	20
			Cheerios	3/4 cup	17
			Milk	1 cup	12
			Banana	1 medium	20
					Total 69
12:30 P.M.	Huma-log	7u	Sub sandwich– 6" turkey, ham, cheese, lettuce, tomato, onions, pickles, mustard	1	46
			Pretzels	2 1/2 oz bag	34
					Total 80
5:00 P.M./Snack	Humalog	2u	Apple	8 oz/1 large	30
7:15 P.M.	Huma-log	9u			
dinner			Macaroni and cheese, prepared with sliced turkey sausage	1 1/2 cups	98
			Broccoli, steamed	1 cup	8
			Fruit cup	3/4 cup	22
					Total 158
10:30 P.M. bedtime	Glargine 22u				

Notes about day:
Went for a walk after dinner.
Blood glucose has gotten low right before bed several times recently.

			Blood glucose results				
Fasting/ before b'fast/ time	After b'fast/ time	Before lunch/ time	After lunch/ time	Before dinner/ time	After dinner/ time	Before bed/ time	Other/ time
92/ 6:30 A.M.	210/ 8:45 A.M.						
		89/ 12:30 P.M.	154/ 2:00 P.M.				
				126/ 7:00 P.M.	205/ 9:00 P.M.		Checked at 11 P.M., felt low, BG = 65

Table 5-6 lists the diabetes medications available today. There will be even more in the future. Find the diabetes medications that you take to learn more about them.

Checking Blood Glucose

To gain the best understanding of the ups and downs of your blood glucose in response to food, activity, stress, and other things in your life, check your blood glucose at various times of the day. And most importantly, record the results. If you don't record the results, the data from which you could learn is lost. The sample form we provided has a space for after-meal blood glucose checks. As you are learning, these results are very important, but most commercial record books don't provide space for these results. After-meal (one and a half to two hours after the time you begin eating) blood glucose checks help you see the impact of the carbohydrate you ate at that meal. Your blood glucose needs to be in target range both before meals and after. The chart on page 7 gives you the target ranges of blood glucose so you can see where yours are in relation to them.

Now don't be alarmed; you don't need to check your blood glucose seven times a day! To observe the ups and downs in your blood glucose, yet avoid feeling like a human pincushion, set up a rotating blood glucose checking pattern. Check your blood glucose two to three times a day at different times on different days. In just a few days, you'll have results from around the clock. Here's a four-day sample pattern with two checks a day:

	Fasting	1–2 hrs after breakfast	Before lunch	1–2 hrs after lunch	Before dinner	1–2 hrs after dinner	Bed	Other
Day 1	■	■						
Day 2			■	■				
Day 3					■	■		
Day 4	■							■

TABLE 5-6   Diabetes Medications

Category	Generic and brand name of medication	Action to control blood glucose	Side effects	Carbohydrate counting
Sulfonylureas	Chlorpropamide (Diabinese) Tolazamide (Tolinase) Tolbutamide (Orinase) Glipizide (Glucotrol, Glucotrol XL), Glyburide (Glynase, DiaBeta, Micronase) Glimepiride (Amaryl)	Helps the pancreas make more insulin. Usually take before a meal once or twice a day. Can combine with metformin, alpha-glucosidase inhibitors, glitazones, or insulin.	Could cause hypoglycemia and weight gain.	Carbohydrate needs to be similar at meals and snacks.
Meglitinides	Repaglinide (Prandin)	Helps pancreas quickly produce insulin to lower blood glucose after eating. Take before meals.	Can cause hypoglycemia if medication is taken but you don't eat or only eat a small amount of carb.	Best if carb content of meals is similar; however, you can learn to adjust the amount of medication for the amount of food you eat at the meal.
D-phenylalanine	Nateglinides (Starlix)	Same as the meglitinides.		

TABLE 5 - 6   Diabetes Medications (continued)

Category	Generic and brand name of medication	Action to control blood glucose	Side effects	Carbohydrate counting
Biguanide	Metformin (Glucophage, Glucophage XR)	Lowers blood glucose by decreasing liver production of glucose and helping the muscles use glucose better. Can combine with sulfonylureas, glitazones, alpha-glucosidase inhibitors, or insulin.	Upset stomach; may lose a few pounds when start taking; do not take if you have kidney or liver disease. Do not take pill if you drink alcohol daily. Does not cause hypoglycemia.	Best if carb content of meals is similar.
Biguanide/ sulfonylureas combination	Glucovance (combination of metformin and glyburide)	Action of biguanide and sulfonylurea.	Can cause hypoglycemia.	Best if carb content of meals is similar.
Glitazones	Rosiglitazone (Avandia) Pioglitazone (Actos)	Helps sensitize your body's tissues to better use the insulin you make. Can combine with sulfonylureas, alpha-glucosidase inhibitors, metformin, or insulin.	Not to be used if you have liver problems. It can interfere with the effectiveness of birth control pills. Does not cause hypoglycemia. Can cause weight gain.	Best if carb content of meals is similar.

Alpha-glucosidase inhibitors	Acarbose (Precose) Miglitol (Glyset)	Slows the breakdown of carbohydrates in the food you eat. Reduces the blood glucose rise after the meal.	Gas, bloating; do not use if there is no carbohydrate in the meal. Does not cause hypoglycemia.	Best if carb content of meals is similar.
Insulin	Rapid-acting: lispro, aspart Short-acting: regular Intermediate-acting: NPH, lente Long-acting: ultralente, glargine (Lantus) Premixed combinations: 70/30, 50/50 (NPH and regular) 75/25 (NPH and lispro) 70/30 (NPH and aspart)	Lowers blood sugar by putting insulin into the body.	Can cause hypoglycemia and weight gain.	Carb content of meals can vary if you learn to adjust insulin based on your insulin:carbohydrate ratio.

Your health care provider can suggest blood glucose checking patterns that help you focus on particular questions you want to answer. Also, you'll likely need to check your blood glucose levels more often when you start Carb Counting. You might also have to check more if you make a change in the dose of medication, add a medication, start an exercise program, etc. When your diabetes plan changes, more blood glucose checks can only be helpful.

If you take insulin several times a day and use Advanced Carb Counting, then you'll need to check your blood glucose levels at least four times a day—when you wake up and before each meal. You need to know your blood glucose level to make a decision about how much insulin you need.

Physical Activity

In almost all cases, being physically active lowers blood glucose. Being physically active is an important part of managing your diabetes as well as an important part of staying healthy and controlling blood lipids and blood pressure. If you are not physically active, think about what you are willing to do to start being so. Perhaps it's a twenty-minute walk two times a week or fifteen minutes on your stationary bike three times a week or simply some more housework or gardening. Don't forget—any physical activity helps!

Use the "other" column or the "notes" section at the bottom to record the type and amount of physical activity you do and when you do them.

Emotions, Stress, Illness, and Unusual Situations

We know that changes in day-to-day events can and do affect blood glucose levels. It's important to record information about your emotions and stressful situations. Illness, medical tests, or surgery can affect your blood glucose. And so can a deadline at work or a heated argument, even if you're just a bystander. It's also important to record positive emotions and situations, too. For example, vacations might be a positive situation, but you eat differently and at different times. You may be well yourself, but you have a sick child or a family emergency. Women should note menstrual periods on the form as well. The various phases of the menstrual cycle, including the hormonal surges of adolescence and menopause, can affect blood glucose levels. You can use the "other" column or "notes" at the bottom for recording these events.

Meet Jane   Jane is a 45-year-old schoolteacher who was recently diagnosed with type 2 diabetes. She takes 500 mg of metformin before breakfast and dinner. She feels she gets enough physical activity at work. She is interested in Basic Carb Counting as a way to keep her blood glucose in control but also have flexibility with the food choices she makes.

She checks her blood glucose when she gets up and does a second check at various times before and after meals. One day she checks after lunch and the next day after dinner but always within one to two hours after she starts to eat. Her blood glucoses after lunch are 140–175 mg/dl, within her target range after meals. But the ones after dinner are in the 200–230 mg/dl range, and she is concerned about this. She looks at the amount of carbs she eats— about 60 g at lunch and 110 g at dinner. She sees that she is not active when she gets home. She fixes dinner and watches her favorite TV shows. But after lunch, she is teaching and on her feet and moving for three more hours.

Keeping records helped Jane learn how the amount of carbs she eats and her activity level has an effect on her blood glucose. She realizes she needs to balance the amount of carb she eats each day by eating more at lunch when she is active and less in the evening. She and the dietitian she is working with set a goal of 45–60 g of carb at lunch and dinner.

You can see Jane's record in Table 5-7 on the next two pages.

T A B L E 5 - 7 Carbohydrate Counting and Blood Glucose Results Record					
Day/Date: _Tuesday, January 23_					
Time/ meal	**Diabetes medicines**		**Food**		**Carb count (servings/ grams)**
	Type	**Amount**	**Type**	**Amount**	
6:00 A.M./ 6:15 A.M./ B'fast	metformin	500 mg	Frozen waffles	2	29
			Maple syrup	2 Tbsp	26
			Raspberries	1/2 cup	8
			Yogurt with fruit, nonfat with low-cal sweetener	1/2 cup	10
					Total 73
12:30 P.M./ Lunch			Chunky split-pea and ham soup	1 11-oz can	33
			Ritz crackers	5	9
			Pear	1 6 oz	22
					Total 64
6:00 P.M./ Dinner	metformin	500 mg	Pork chop–baked	3 oz	0
			Mashed potatoes	1 cup	33
			with butter	1 tsp	0
			Green peas	1/2 cup	15
			Dinner roll	1	15
			with butter	1 tsp	0
			Apple pie	1/8 9" pie	43
					Total 106
Notes about day: On my feet and moving while teaching after lunch for 3 hours.					

Blood glucose results

Fasting/ before b'fast/ time	After b'fast/ time	Before lunch/ time	After lunch/ time	Before dinner/ time	After dinner/ time	Before bed/ time	Other/ time
90/ 6:00 A.M.							
			165/ 2:00 P.M.				
				116/ 6:00 P.M.	223/ 8:00 P.M.		

6

Protein, Fat, and Alcohol Count, Too

True, the focus of Carbohydrate Counting is on the foods that contain carbohydrate. It's also true that the protein and fat in foods, when you eat them in recommended and reasonable amounts, have little effect on blood glucose levels. However, you cannot ignore the foods that contain protein and fat. Here are the reasons why:

1. Protein and fat have calories and unfortunately all calories do count. Protein and fat might not affect your blood glucose levels much, but if you eat too much, they can add to your waistline. Examples of high-fat foods are salad dressings, margarine, mayonnaise, and cream cheese. Most foods with protein contain some fat. The amount of fat varies from very little—such as in fish like flounder or sole, or chicken breasts—to a lot—such as in nuts, prime rib, cheese, and sausage. It's important to keep in mind that fats, no matter whether they are healthier fat or not-so-healthy fat, are concentrated sources of calories. And they literally often get lost in the sauce—in other words, you are eating them, but you don't really see them. Think about margarine on vegetables or salad dressing on salad.

2. Too much protein, especially animal protein, and too much fat, especially saturated fat, are not healthy for anyone—but especially for people with diabetes. Learn more in this chapter.

3. Fat and protein in your meal may slow down the rise in blood glucose. When you eat a meal that is higher in protein than usual—for example, you enjoy an 8-oz steak or prime rib—your blood glucose might rise more slowly than you expect. In addition, when you eat a meal that is higher in fat than usual—for example, fried chicken, mashed potatoes, and gravy followed by a piece of cheesecake for dessert—your blood glucose might rise more slowly and peak later than you expect. You need to know about these differences and account for them as you manage your blood glucose levels.

The Need for Protein and Fat

Our bodies need some protein to build muscles. Protein is made up of amino acids—the building blocks of protein—that the body needs in order to work. Interestingly, several amino acids can be converted into glucose. This glucose can then enter the bloodstream and be used for energy.

Our bodies also need some fat, but only a small amount and in the healthy varieties. Fat carries the fat-soluble vitamins A, D, E, and K. A couple of so-called "essential" fats must be in the foods you eat because the body can't make them. Fats supply energy, cushion the body's vital organs, and provide insulation to keep us warm. Also, fat is well known for making food taste good.

WHICH FOODS CONTAIN PROTEIN?

Many people would answer "red meat, poultry, and seafood," which is correct. But actually protein turns up in other food groups, too. Eggs and cheese are also rich sources of protein. Foods from other food groups contain protein in combination with carbohydrate, such as dried beans and peas, grains, and vegetables. Then there are nuts, which contain protein and a lot of fat—albeit healthier fats. On average, an ounce (oz) of protein-rich food contains 7 grams (g) of protein. As noted, the fat per ounce in these foods can vary from none to a high of about 8 g.

WHICH FOODS CONTAIN FAT?

Some foods are just about 100% fat, such as butter, margarine, or regular salad dressing. They are often added to other foods to make them taste better. You might call these "added fats." On average, these contain about 5 g of fat and 45 calories per serving. Plenty of foods contain zero fat, such as pasta, broccoli, and lettuce—that is until you add fat when you cook them or slather fat on at the table. Other foods contain some, but not all, of their calories as fat, such as meats, cheese, nuts, whole-milk dairy foods, and most desserts. You might call these "attached fats," where fat is naturally part of the food.

Fats in foods are actually combinations of different types of fatty acids. In foods, the fat is made up of varying amounts of three types of fat—saturated, polyunsaturated, and monounsaturated. Since you've likely heard a lot about trans fats, you might wonder why we haven't mentioned them as a type of fat. That's because they are considered a saturated fat. We'll talk more about trans fats below.

Following are lists of the three different fats, how they act in the body, and a few example foods that contain a majority of their fat from the mentioned type.

MONOUNSATURATED FATS

ACTIONS: LOWER TOTAL CHOLESTEROL, LDL AND HDL

- Oils (liquid canola, olive, peanut)
- Olives
- Nuts

POLYUNSATURATED FATS

There are two types of polyunsaturated fats—omega-3s and omega-6s.

Actions of omega-3s: Lower risk for heart disease by decreasing stickiness of blood platelets and lowering triglycerides.

- Fatty fish, such as salmon, sardines, herring, and albacore tuna

- Flax (ground) and flax seed oil, soybean, and canola oil

- Walnuts

Actions of omega-6s: Lower total cholesterol and LDL. They also lower HDL, which isn't a benefit.

- Oils (liquid corn, safflower, soybean)

SATURATED FATS

Action: Raise total and LDL cholesterol

- Meats, poultry, seafood
- Butter
- Cream cheese
- Whole-milk dairy foods

Trans Fats Defined

Some trans fats are found naturally in foods such as meats and dairy foods. Some trans fats are created through a food process called partial hydrogenation. Partial hydrogenation takes an unsaturated fat and makes it saturated—or solid. Think of a margarine made from liquid corn oil formed into a stick. Food manufacturers use partial hydrogenation to create the more solid form of fat and increase the shelf life of products. Today, Americans get about 2–4% of our calories from trans fats, which doesn't sound like much, but is enough to cause concern. Why? Because research shows that even small amounts of trans fats, such as other saturated fats, raise LDL cholesterol. In addition, they also lower HDLs, which is not good.

To limit your intake of trans fats:

▓ Lower your total fat and saturated fat intake.

▓ Limit your intake of foods with partially hydrogenated fat, such as margarine, cookies, crackers, fried snack foods, frozen convenience foods, and fried restaurant foods.

▓ Take advantage of new foods that are trans fat free, such as newer margarines and salad dressings.

▓ Watch the Nutrition Facts panel—before or by January 2006, food manufacturers will have to provide information about trans fats under the fat information. Some manufacturers are already providing this.

WHAT DOES PROTEIN DO TO BLOOD GLUCOSE?

For many years it was thought that 50% of the protein we ate was converted into glucose and that protein just raised blood glucose more slowly than carbohydrate. This theory encouraged health care providers to teach people with diabetes to always eat protein in combination with carbohydrate. Newer research throws doubt on this theory. Recent studies have shown that protein stimulates the production of some insulin in people with type 2 diabetes and that this small rise in insulin actually lowers blood glucose. In people with type 1 diabetes, protein has little effect on blood glucose, unless very large portions are eaten. Unfortunately, large portions of protein can increase blood glucose and cause a need for more insulin or other diabetes medication.

So, what's the advice about protein today? Monitor your blood glucose and see what works best for you. Some people feel they have better blood glucose control and have greater satiety and less hunger between meals with some protein at each meal. Other people feel that protein in a bedtime snack is helpful if they use a bedtime snack. Still others don't think the added protein makes a difference. As you aim to spread your protein throughout your day, remember that the amounts that are recommended are relatively small. Also keep in mind that a portion of protein-rich food or "meat" is about 3 oz cooked.

It is true that a high-protein meal—which often is high in both protein and fat—may delay the rise of blood glucose. In other words, the high amount of protein and fat slow down the rise of blood glucose from the carbohydrate in the meal. This may be due, in part, to a delay in stomach emptying. If you are used to eating a 3- to 4-oz serving of meat at dinner and then on a rare occasion you eat an 8-oz sirloin, you might find that when you check your blood glucose level one to two hours later, it's not as high as you thought it would be. Then if you check it three to four hours later, when you thought it would be headed down, it is higher than you expected. There are various ways to manage this situation (see chapter 13) when it happens on occasion. However, keep in mind that it is healthiest to eat small amounts of protein and fat.

Meet Jan   Jan has type 1 diabetes. She takes four shots of insulin a day—one shot of glargine (Lantus) at bedtime and rapid-acting lispro before meals (see Table 6-1). She has had the experience of eating a meal high in protein and fat and finding that her blood glucose is not as high as she expected two hours after she started eating. This evening she decided that she was going to check her blood glucose more often to determine the effect of a high-protein and high-fat meal. She'll take them to her health care provider to talk about strategies to deal with this situation. She thinks she might need to take her lispro insulin in the middle or at the end of the meal to better control the delayed rise in blood glucose level.

Meet Eric   Eric has type 2 diabetes, is overweight, and is quite insulin resistant. He takes metformin before breakfast and dinner and takes Prandin,

TABLE 6 - 1 Jan's Record: High-Protein, High-Fat Meal (Person with type 1 diabetes)

Day/Date: *Tuesday, January 23*

Time/meal	Diabetes medicines		Food		Carb count (servings/grams)	Blood glucose results			
	Type	Amount	Type	Amount		Before dinner (7 P.M.)	2 hours (9 P.M.)	3 hours (10 P.M.)	Bedtime (11 P.M.)
7 P.M.	Humalog	6 units	Sirloin steak	8 oz		107	155	261	143
			Baked potato with	6 oz	2/30 g				
			Sour cream	2 Tbsp					
			Butter	2 tsp					
			Salad bar with	1 trip	2/30 g				
			Thousand Island dressing	3 Tbsp	0.5/7 g				
			Dinner roll	1 medium	1/15 g				
			Butter	1 tsp					
			Strawberry shortcake	1/2 portion	2/35 g				
			Total		8/117 g				

a rapid-acting diabetes pill, before his three meals. He decided to check his blood glucose levels a number of times after eating a rather high-protein and high-fat meal. He wanted to learn what this type of meal and foods did to his blood glucose (see Table 6-2). Then with his chart in hand, he talked to his health care provider about the possibility of increasing his dose of Prandin for a meal like this. However, he recognizes very well that doing this on a regular basis would probably make him gain weight and not do much for his arteries either.

His health care provider also mentioned that certain foods, pizza being one of them, can have a delayed and somewhat unpredictable effect on blood glucose levels (see Table 6-3).

It is important to note that the impact of eating larger than usual amounts of protein and fat varies from person to person and varies according to each person's diabetes management plan. The best advice is to monitor your blood glucose several times in the hours after you eat meals or foods that are higher in protein and fat. For instance, you might want to check your blood glucose both two hours and three hours after the meal rather than just two hours after. At two hours you might not have seen the full impact of the meal on your blood glucose level. Learn how your body responds to these meals so you can determine a plan to manage them.

To learn more ways to manage these situations, you may also want to read the section in chapter 13, "When to Take Mealtime Insulin—Before, During, or After?" on page 183.

WHAT IS IMPORTANT ABOUT PROTEIN AND DIABETES?

The current American Diabetes Association (ADA) nutrition recommendations suggest that people with diabetes get 10–20% of their daily calories from protein. You can get the protein you need from either animal sources, such as poultry, dairy foods, and red meat, or from vegetable sources, such as grains, beans, legumes, low-fat dairy foods, and vegetables.

TABLE 6 - 2 Eric's Record: High-Protein, High-Fat Meal (Person with type 2 diabetes/insulin resistance)

Day/Date: *Tuesday, January 23*

| Time/meal | Diabetes medicines | | Food | | Carb count (servings/grams) | Blood glucose results | | | | |
	Type	Amount	Type	Amount		Before dinner (7 P.M.)	2 hours (9 P.M.)	3 hours (10 P.M.)	Bedtime (11 P.M.)
7 P.M.	Metformin	850 mg	Sirloin steak	8 oz		147	198	280	223
			Baked potato with	6 oz	2/30 g				
			Sour cream	2 Tbsp					
			Butter	2 tsp					
			Salad bar with	1 trip	2/30 g				
			Thousand Island dressing	3 Tbsp	0.5/7 g				
			Dinner roll	1 medium	1/15 g				
			Butter	1 tsp					
			Strawberry shortcake	1/2 portion	2/35 g				
			Total		8/117 g				

TABLE 6 - 3 Sample Record: Effect of Pizza on Blood Glucose Level

Day/Date: *Tuesday, January 23*

Time/meal	Diabetes medicines		Food		Carb count (servings/grams)	Blood glucose results				
	Type	Amount	Type	Amount		Before lunch (noon)	1 hour (1 P.M.)	2 hours (2 P.M.)	3 hours (3 P.M.)	
12:00 noon	Humalog	4 units	Pizza with extra cheese, pepperoni, and onions (regular crust)	3 medium slices	6/92 g	117	178	192	234	
			Garden salad with Light Italian dressing	1 1/2 cups 2 Tbsp	0/5 g 0/2 g					
			Total		6/99 g					

You may need to consider lowering your intake of protein if you are diagnosed with diabetic kidney disease. However, there is even stronger evidence that controlling blood glucose and blood pressure does more to prevent and/or delay the progression of diabetic kidney disease. The ADA suggests that your health care provider measure your kidney function each year, because the best way to prevent the progression of kidney disease is early detection and management. Kidney function can be measured by a spot urine test. If you have evidence that you are spilling protein, which indicates some kidney damage, then your health care provider may suggest you do a 24-hour urine collection.

HOW MUCH PROTEIN SHOULD YOU EAT?

Whether you follow the ADA guideline of 10–20% of calories or the U.S. Government recommended daily amount (RDA) for protein, which is slightly lower, you may need to trim down your portions of protein. The RDA for the average male is about 60–65 g of protein and for the average female about 50–55 g of protein. If we translate this into servings of protein, that's two to three (3-oz) servings of cooked meat or meat substitutes per day. If you have evidence of diabetic kidney disease, you may be encouraged to eat no more than this amount of protein. And there is some evidence that eating more vegetable protein foods, such as soy products or legumes, rather than animal protein foods, may be less damaging to your kidneys.

Like we said above, each ounce of protein food contains about 7 g of protein. So, a 2-oz serving of protein has 14 g of protein and a 3-oz servings has 21 g. The serving size of protein for your meal plan is usually 2–3 oz of cooked protein. That is a piece of meat about the size of the palm of your hand. While an ounce of meat has 7 g of protein, the differences in choices of meat decide the amount of fat in the serving (see Table 6-4). The more fat, the more calories you get, too.

TABLE 6-4 The Differences in Meat Servings		
Type of meat (3 oz cooked)	Fat (g)	Calories
Very lean meats (white meat chicken, flounder)	0–1	105
Lean meat (tenderloin, dark meat chicken)	9	165
Medium-fat meats (ground beef, pork chops)	15	225
High-fat meats (country pork ribs, regular cheese)	24	300

WHAT IS IMPORTANT ABOUT FAT AND DIABETES?

When you have diabetes, you have an increased risk of developing heart disease. That includes heart attacks, strokes, high blood pressure, and related circulatory problems. In fact, people with type 2 diabetes have two to four times greater risk of developing heart disease than people without diabetes. One problem is that many people with diabetes, particularly people with type 2 diabetes, have abnormal blood fat levels. Typically, that's low HDL cholesterol and high triglyceride levels. Many people with type 2 diabetes have an LDL that is not that elevated. However, it is now known that though the LDL is not that elevated, the type of fat particles are more likely to be of the small, dense type. This is especially true if triglycerides are elevated. This type of LDL may increase the appearance of heart disease. The goal for LDL cholesterol is 100 mg/dl or less.

The risk of heart disease is the reason for one of the strongest diabetes nutrition recommendations: Eat less saturated fat. There are some quick ways to eat less saturated fat, total fat, and cholesterol:

- Choose lean, reduced-fat, low-fat, or fat-free foods. (Watch the carb content of these foods.)

- Prepare foods in low-fat ways.

- Eat small portions.

Today there are many leaner cuts of meat, skinless chicken and turkey parts, reduced-fat cheeses, fat-free milk, and other lower-

T A B L E 6 - 5 Blood Fat Goals with Diabetes*	
LDL ("bad" cholesterol)	<100 mg/dl**
HDL ("good" cholesterol)	>40 mg/dl (men), >50 mg/dl (women)
Triglycerides	<150 mg/dl

* Note the ADA recommendations for people with diabetes are slightly different from those for the general population without heart disease.
** ADA recommends that if LDL is greater than 130 mg/dl, that medication to lower LDL (a statin medication) be started immediately.

fat dairy foods to make your job of reducing saturated fat and cholesterol easier.

To determine how much fat and what types of fat to eat, you need to know whether your blood fat levels are normal (see Table 6-5). The ADA recommends that adults with diabetes have their blood fats checked every year.

If you are at a healthy weight and have normal blood fat levels, you can eat 30% of your calories from fat, but saturated fat should not account for more than 10% of your total calories. You want to keep polyunsaturated fats at or below 10% of your calories, too. Monounsaturated fats can be in the range of 10–15% of calories. Try to eat no more than 300 mg of cholesterol per day. If you have high triglycerides, then lower your carbohydrate intake to about 40% of calories and increase your total fat calories to about 40% with monounsaturated fats contributing about 20% of those calories (this is, by the way, easier said than done for most people). Don't let all these percentages confuse you. Review Table 2-3 in chapter 2 (pages 28–29) and ask a dietitian for help.

WHAT CAN YOU LEARN FROM THE GRAMS OF TOTAL FAT?

Are you a little curious about how you can figure how much total fat and the types of fats you need? Here's an example using a meal plan that calls for 1500 daily calories with 30% coming from fat.

Total number of calories: 1500

Multiply calories by 30%:   1500
                             $\times .30$
                             450 calories from fat

Since there are 9 calories per gram of fat, divide calories from fat by 9:

$$\frac{450}{9} = 50 \text{ g of total fat}$$

Therefore, this meal plan suggests you eat under 50 g of fat per day. Now you can also figure the number of grams of saturated and polyunsaturated fat to eat so you can stay under 10% for each.

Multiply calories by 10%:   1500
                             $\times .10$
                             150 calories from fat

Divide this number by 9 (9 calories per gram of fat):

$$\frac{150}{9} = 17 \text{ g of saturated}$$
and 17 g of poly-
unsaturated fat

You can figure the number of grams of monounsaturated fat to eat for 10–15% of your daily calories. You already know that 10% of 1500 calories is 17 g of fat. But to find the number of grams of monounsaturated fat in 15% of the 1500 calories you would:

Multiply calories by 15%:   1500
                             $\times .15$
                             225 calories from fat

Divide this number by 9 (9 calories per gram of fat):

$$\frac{225}{9} = 25 \text{ g of mono-unsaturated fat}$$

DO FAT REPLACERS CONTAIN CARBOHYDRATE?

The push to eat less fat has given rise to a flurry of reduced-fat, low-fat, and fat-free foods. When fat is removed from food to lower the fat content and calories, food manufacturers have to put something into the products to make them continue to taste good. Using ingredients that are called "fat replacers," manufacturers can make reduced-fat, low-fat, and fat-free foods, such as ice cream, sour cream, cream cheese, salad dressing, potato chips, and margarine. Fat replacers are ingredients that are made from carbohydrate, protein, or fat. An example of a carbohydrate-based fat replacer is maltodextrin, a modified food starch. An example of a fat-based fat replacer is olestra. The majority of fat replacers in use today are made of carbohydrate. When the fat is taken out and these fat replacers are put in, the calories are usually, but not always, lower. But the carbohydrate content usually is higher.

For people with diabetes these extra grams of carbohydrate can certainly affect your blood glucose levels. In the supermarket read the Total Carbohydrate on the Nutrition Facts labels on reduced-fat, low-fat, and fat-free foods to determine their carb count. Try a few. Find ones that you enjoy and help you achieve your nutrition goals. If you don't like the taste of one, try another or don't use these foods. There are other ways to lower your fat intake.

ALCOHOL

True, alcohol is not food, but it does contain calories, and some beverages, such as regular beer, contain carbohydrate. The calories in most alcoholic drinks—distilled spirits and wine—are from alcohol. The calories from alcohol are actually more concentrated than carbohydrates. Alcohol has seven calories per gram versus the four in carbohydrate. (Fat provides nine calories per gram.) So, the calories from alcohol can add up quickly. The most important general message about alcohol is "drink in moderation." The U.S. Government defines this as one drink a day for women and two drinks a day for men. What's the amount of "one drink"? Look on page 227 in Appendix 1. You might consider this a lot of alcohol. One health benefit has been associated with alcohol intake—an increase in the HDL, or good, cholesterol. However, if you don't currently drink, this is not a reason to start now.

Alcohol is interesting in that it can do opposite things—it can both lower blood glucose levels and raise blood glucose levels. Let's look first at how it can lower blood glucose levels, because that is of greater concern.

Alcohol Can Lower Blood Glucose

Firstly, the calories from alcohol will not convert to glucose and raise blood glucose. Secondly, alcohol can decrease the amount of glucose that is put out from the liver. If alcohol is doing this in your body and you have taken insulin or an oral diabetes medicine that can cause low blood glucose, this can produce a double whammy effect. The liver will not produce glucose to raise your blood glucose and you'll develop hypoglycemia if you drink alcohol and don't eat. When you drink alcohol and take a blood glucose lowering medication, eating a sufficient amount of food is the key to avoiding alcohol-induced hypoglycemia. People can particularly have problems with low blood glucose from alcohol a number of hours after drinking and/or overnight.

Drink Alcohol Safely—The How To's:

1. Know your blood glucose. Don't drink if your blood glucose is too low.

2. Eat carbohydrate-containing food that will raise your blood glucose and prevent low blood glucose before, during, and/or after you drink.

3. If you drink in the evening, check your blood glucose before you go to bed. If it seems to be decreasing, have some carb-containing food.

4. If you drink alcohol that does contain carbohydrate, such as regular beer; mixed drinks with fruit juice, soda, or other carbohydrate-containing ingredients; or liqueur, count these grams of carb as part of your carb allotment. However, if your blood glucose tends to spiral down with alcohol or you are just moving to more intensive diabetes management and you're not quite comfortable covering the carb from alcohol, just consider the carb from alcoholic drinks as extra carb.

5. Clearly, doing blood glucose checks and keeping track of how much and what you drink will help you learn your body's reaction to alcohol.

6. The most important message is to drink in moderation and responsibly.

Alcohol Can Cause High Blood Glucose

Blood glucose can also go too high with alcoholic beverages. That's because some alcoholic beverages, as noted above, do contain carbohydrate. It's not the alcohol causing the rise in blood glucose; it's the carbohydrate.

Look in Appendix 1 , which lists various types of alcohol with the serving sizes and grams of carbohydrate.

7

Weigh and Measure Foods
A KEY TO YOUR SUCCESS

You can eat only "healthy foods" and still gain weight. Healthy foods—such as whole-grain breads and cereals, fruits, and vegetables—do contain calories and it's possible to eat too much of them. Bottom line: It's not just a matter of *what* you eat, it's clearly also a matter of *how much*.

Surprisingly, the extra carbohydrate from servings that are just a bit too large can add up quickly. Perhaps you regularly eat an extra 1/2 cup of pasta or potatoes at dinner—an extra 15 grams (g) of carb—or a large apple rather than a medium apple at lunch—about 10 g extra carb. And, it's not just the carbohydrate. It might be an extra ounce or two of meat (protein and fat) at dinner and an extra tablespoon of regular salad dressing (fat) at lunch. It is easy to tell yourself that these extras are too small to keep you from achieving blood glucose control or your other diabetes goals. After all, you're not eating a candy bar or slice of cheesecake! That is true, but extra servings on a daily basis can mean the difference between hitting your blood glucose targets—and/or losing weight—and not.

Our Super-sized Society

In this society, it is a huge (literally!) challenge to eat only the portion sizes we really need, with ever-larger dinner plates, super-sized fast food meals, and all-you-can-eat buffet restaurants. For example, in a fast food restaurant, the difference in calories between a "value meal" and a "super-sized value meal" is 600 calories! Unfortunately, we've lost sight of reasonable portions. This is especially true if you frequently go to restaurants where common serving sizes are a 10-ounce (oz) steak, 2 cups of pasta, a three-egg omelet, or a jumbo order of French fries. Clearly, these typical restaurant portions don't follow the serving sizes that we see on food Nutrition Facts labels or the servings suggested in this book. Unfortunately, these super-sized servings are one of several reasons why today 65% of Americans are overweight or obese, 15% of children and adolescents are overweight, and we have an epidemic of type 2 diabetes in which people are being diagnosed at younger and younger ages.

What Size Serving?

It is likely that you already have all the tools you need to pinpoint the size of your servings. Do you have measuring spoons and measuring cups for liquids and solids? Most every household has these valuable kitchen utensils, but they might be hidden away. Find them a new home—up front on the shelf nearest to the dishes that you use. You will use these tools at every meal for a while. Table

TABLE 7-1   Common Household Measurements
3 teaspoons (tsp) = 1 tablespoon (Tbsp)
4 Tbsp = 1/4 cup = 2 fluid ounces
8 Tbsp = 1/2 cup = 4 fluid ounces
16 Tbsp = 1 cup = 8 fluid ounces
1 cup = 1/2 pint
2 cups = 1 pint
1 ounce = 30 grams (dry)

7-1 can help you get comfortable with the weights and measures you'll be seeing often.

Here's what you need:

Measuring spoons. A set of measuring spoons with 1/2 teaspoon (tsp), 1 tsp, 1/2 tablespoon (Tbsp), and 1 Tbsp. When you use these measuring spoons, you'll see that there are 3 tsp in 1 Tbsp. Don't use your regular silverware for measuring foods. They vary in size based on style and won't give you exact measurements.

Measuring cup—liquids. A 1- or 2-cup measuring cup with lines showing 1/4-, 1/3-, 1/2-, 2/3-, and 3/4-cup measures. A liquid measuring cup should be clear (glass or plastic) so you can see through it. To measure liquids correctly, set the cup down and bend down at eye level to make sure the liquid reaches the proper line.

Measuring cup—solids. A set of 1/4-, 1/2-, 3/4-, and 1-cup measuring cups. Choose the correct size for your serving, for example, of cereal or rice, and fill it to the top. Level it with the flat edge of a knife. For instance, if you need 1/2 cup of uncooked hot cereal, measure it in a 1/2-cup measure and level it off with a flat knife to eliminate any excess.

Food scale. Get at least an inexpensive ($5–$15) food scale. You will mainly use it to measure foods that you measure in ounces, such as fresh fruit or bagels, potatoes, snack foods, cereals, baked goods, meats, fish, and cheese.

Upscale food scales? More expensive scales are available, but they are not necessary. You can spend a low of $25 to a high of $190. On the low end, the food scale measures ounces, pounds, grams, and kilograms. On the high end are digital scales that give you an exact measure with a numeric digital readout rather than making you read between the lines. And there are scales that actually give you the gram weight of the food and the grams of carbohydrate in that amount of the food for about $400. There are many scales available on *www.amazon.com*, or do an online search for food scales and you'll find many options.

Eyes. Don't underestimate a well-trained and honest set of eyes. Your eyes are an invaluable measuring tool because you always have them with you.

Specialized items. A product called the *Portion Doctor Kit,* which has been developed by a creative dietitian, may be a helpful resource if you are just getting started with portion control and/or particularly have a difficult time controlling your portions. The kit includes four clear glass items—two plates, one bowl, and one drinking glass. It also comes with an instructional guidebook. To learn more about it or purchase it, go to *www.portiondoctor.com.*

Nutrition Facts label. The Nutrition Facts label on most packaged foods today is one of your best tools because it must list the serving size. Best yet, it's free and widely available. The serving sizes on food labels today are regulated by the FDA. These are the serving sizes that food manufacturers must use to comply with the food-labeling law. For us consumers, this is good news. Additionally, all the packaged food manufacturers are using the same sizes of servings. This means that one serving of dry cereal is 30 g or about 1 oz for all dry cereals on the market. (Take care not to confuse the weight in grams listed next to the serving size with the grams of carbohydrate in one serving listed near Total Carbohydrates. Those are two different numbers.) Another helpful addition to the Nutrition Facts is the serving size in "common household terms," such as 7 crackers or 2/3 cup. That makes serving sizes easier to understand.

All the nutrition information on the Nutrition Facts label is based on one serving. Use the serving sizes to help you learn what reasonable portions are. If you usually eat a larger quantity of that food, perhaps your portions are too large or the portion you may be counting as one serving is actually two or three.

It is important to say here that the food label serving size is not necessarily the same as a serving for Carb Counting. When it comes to foods that contain carbohydrate, remember the number 15. If you are counting servings, one serving of a carbohydrate food has about 15 g of carbohydrate. For example, look at the

Nutrition Facts panel for a cold cereal on page 100. It says a 1 cup serving is 49 g of carbohydrate. When you divide 49 by 15, you see that this serving is 3 carbohydrate servings with 4 g of carbohydrate left over. So, a serving of 1 cup of this cereal is a little over 3 carbohydrate servings. If you are counting carbohydrate by grams, you just check the serving size and grams of total carbohydrate on the label and make sure your serving size is the same. Or you adjust your carb count for the size of the serving you eat.

The Nutrition Facts panel is an excellent resource for learning about the carbohydrate content of foods. Nearly all Nutrition Facts labels provide the grams of Total Carbohydrate. Chapter 8 is all about what's on the food label and how to use it.

When to Weigh and Measure

It is particularly important to weigh and measure your foods as you begin to count carbohydrates. If you weigh and measure all your foods and beverages for a couple of weeks, you will learn a lot about the correct serving size and maybe some surprising facts about your usual serving size. Don't worry; you do not have to weigh and measure foods every day for years to come! That's not practical or realistic, especially when you eat away from home. Keep in mind, however, that the more often you practice weighing and measuring foods and beverages at home, the easier it is to estimate correct servings when you eat away from home.

Always weigh or measure new foods. Occasionally weigh or measure foods and beverages you regularly eat to check that your eyes are still seeing correct serving sizes—those portions can slowly grow over time. Another time to go back to weighing and measuring foods is when you see your blood glucose levels or your weight start to climb. Perhaps one reason these numbers are on the rise is that your portions have grown. The bottom line for mastering serving sizes is honesty. If you are honest with yourself, your servings will be on the money more times than not.

Learn more tips and tricks to estimate portions when you eat away from home in chapter 10.

Tips and Tricks

To help you estimate servings, here are some "handy" guides.

- Thumb tip (from first knuckle) = 1 tsp
  Example: 1 tsp mayonnaise or margarine

- Thumb (whole—to second knuckle) = 1 Tbsp
  Example: 1 Tbsp salad dressing or cream cheese

- Two fingers lengthwise = 1 oz
  Example: 1 oz cheese or meat

- Palm of hand = 3 oz
  Example: 3 oz boneless cooked meat (a regular size deck of cards or a bar of soap are also good examples)

- Tight fist = 1/2 cup
  Example: 1 serving noodles or rice, 1 serving canned fruit

- Loose fist/Cupped hand = 1 cup
  Example: 1 cup vegetables or pasta

These guidelines hold true for most women's hands, but some men's hands are much larger. Check it out for yourself!

At home, always serve meals in the same size plates, glasses, and bowls. This technique helps you judge correct portions, and you don't have to use the measuring tools so often. For instance, use the same glass each time you drink milk. Measure your serving into a measuring cup once or twice. Pour it into the glass. See where your serving comes to in the glass. You can mark it if you want with an indelible marker or piece of masking tape. Every now and then, measure your serving in a measuring cup to check your accuracy. You need to see how much room 1 cup of pasta takes on a dinner plate, 1/2 cup of hot oatmeal in a bowl, and so on. Keep these "pictures" in your mind.

Once you feel confident that you can eyeball serving sizes correctly and honestly, you don't have to weigh and measure everything. It's wise to do so from time to time, perhaps once a week on

Monday, just to make sure your eyes don't lose the "pictures" over time. You can quiz yourself occasionally. Pour the amount of dry cereal, pasta, or rice you usually eat into the container in which you eat it. Then measure the quantity you poured. Is the serving size correct? If not, you can readjust your eyes by using the measuring tools for a week or two.

If you serve family style meals—that means filling large serving bowls and putting them on the table for everyone to help themselves—stop! This style of serving food promotes overeating! Seconds are that much closer to your fork and lips. Begin to serve in the kitchen. If people want seconds, they have to walk for them. If no one needs seconds, wrap them up before you begin to eat.

When you purchase fresh produce (fruits and vegetables) take advantage of the food scales that hang in the market produce area. Weigh individual pieces of fruit. Focus on what a 4-oz banana, 6 1/2-oz orange, or 3 1/2-oz kiwi really looks like. These all represent 1 carbohydrate serving or 15 g of carbohydrate. Think about your shopping and eating habits. Do you reach for the largest apple or banana and count it as 1 serving (15 g) of carbohydrate, but it's really 1 1/2 carb servings (22 g) of carbohydrate or even 2 carb choices (30 g) of carbohydrate? Many of the apples in today's supermarkets are 7–8 oz. Measure pieces of fruit on the food scale in the produce area on several shopping trips. This will help cement a visual picture in your mind of the correct serving of fruit. Then buy the pieces of food that fit your needs on each shopping trip or realize that a half a piece is closer to the serving you need. To keep yourself in check, weigh your produce on occasion to make sure your "pictures" are still sharp. Note that the weights listed for one serving of fresh fruits in Carb Counting food lists include the skin, core, seeds, and rind.

It's so easy to go overboard on servings of meat, poultry, and cheese because one more ounce does not look like that much more. However, it adds another 35–100 calories, depending on the fat content, for each extra ounce. Try this: When you buy a package of cheese, cold cuts, or anything you buy by the ounce, glance at the ounces on the label. Then visualize what 1, 2, or 3 oz looks like. If you buy cheese or cold cuts sliced to order, think about how many meals you will make from that quantity. Let that be your guide to how many ounces you buy. If you make a smoked turkey and Swiss cheese sandwich for lunch with 2 oz of turkey and 1 oz of cheese, how many sandwiches are you going to make until the next time you shop? Buy the amount you need, not just any amount. Another benefit is that you waste less food.

When you purchase a piece of meat, such as pork roast, leg of lamb, or chicken breasts, estimate the amount of raw meat you need to buy. Think about how many people you are feeding, what quantity you will lose in cooking (see the rule of thumb on page 97), and how much you want for leftovers. That's your number. Write it by the item on your shopping list or do your calculations at the meat counter.

Meet Rita

Rita has been overweight for a number of years now. She is 52 and about a year ago found out that she has type 2 diabetes. Her nurse practitioner put her on a diabetes medication that initially helped lower her blood glucose levels, but eventually, she put on another 12 pounds rather than losing weight. Every time Rita came to see the nurse practitioner, she advised Rita to eat less and exercise more. Each time Rita returned, the scale would show a few more pounds—she was up to 183 pounds. That was the most she had ever weighed and was way too much on her 5′4″ frame. She was frustrated and didn't feel like she could get her diabetes in control. The nurse practitioner suggested she see a dietitian. When she made the appointment, the receptionist said she would send her forms and that she should keep food records for the two weeks before she sees the dietitian. She was also encouraged to bring her meter and blood glucose monitoring records for her visit.

Rita came to see the dietitian with all her records in hand. During their session, the dietitian reviewed Rita's food records with her. The dietitian noted that Rita just wrote down the types of

RAW TO COOKED: RULES OF THUMB

Raw meat with no bone: 4 oz raw to get 3 oz cooked.

Raw meat with bone: 5 oz raw to get 3 oz cooked.

Raw poultry with skin: 4 1/4 to 4 1/2 oz to get 3 oz cooked. The extra 1/4 to 1/2 oz accounts for the skin. (Remove the skin before or after cooking.)

Here is an example for a whole chicken: Each family member needs about 3 oz cooked chicken. There are five family members. The chicken has bones and skin, so you need to figure about 5 1/2 oz per person. So, 5 × 5 1/2 = 28 oz or about 1 3/4 pounds. If you want enough for two meals, you need about 3 1/2 pounds. Do not forget a few ounces for the organs stuffed in the cavity. So, you need about a 4-pound chicken.

foods she ate, but not the amounts. It was clear that Rita was, generally speaking, choosing healthy foods to eat. When the dietitian asked Rita if she weighed or measured her foods, Rita said she didn't think it was necessary if she was eating healthy foods and watching her fat intake. The dietitian pointed out that because Rita has to count her calories to lose some weight, she would do better if she weighed and measured her foods as often as possible, especially when she eats at home.

The dietitian began to teach Rita Basic Carb Counting and encouraged her to choose 3 servings of carbohydrate at breakfast, 4 at lunch, and 4 at dinner. The dietitian showed Rita some food models of the serving sizes she should eat. Rita was amazed at how small the portions looked. The dietitian asked Rita what measuring tools she had at home. Rita said she has measuring cups and spoons but doesn't have a food scale. The dietitian encouraged Rita to use her measuring tools and to purchase a $5–$15 food scale. She noted it was particularly important for Rita to measure foods like pasta, dry cereal, rice, potatoes, and milk. Since Rita had been going a bit wild on fresh fruit, the dietitian discussed reasonable servings of these foods. The dietitian encouraged Rita to look for smaller pieces of fruit or to cut a piece of fruit in half.

Rita left the dietitian's office both pleased and disappointed. She was pleased that they identified her servings as a problem area. She believes that if she watches her portions more carefully, she will lose weight and get her blood glucose levels into better control. But she was disappointed because she knows she cannot eat as much as she has been eating.

Rita went back to see the dietitian four weeks later. She brought along her carbohydrate counts and blood glucose results record that the dietitian asked her to keep. This time she had filled in the amounts of the foods she ate. She was pleased because her weight was down 1 1/2 pounds. No longer on the rise! And her blood glucose results had inched down as well. She says that since she has been weighing and measuring her foods, she laughs as she realizes how much she was eating. She believes she can continue to lose weight if she continues to be honest about how much she eats. The dietitian suggested that Rita add some physical activity to her schedule. They discussed what activity Rita was willing to do. She noted that even a small amount of activity each day would help burn calories and lower blood glucose. Rita is going to try to do more gardening this summer and to take a fifteen-minute walk two to three evenings a week.

Rita came back for a third visit two months later with her records in hand. She was scheduled to see both her nurse practitioner and dietitian. Sure enough, she got on the scale, and it showed a weight loss of 4 pounds over two months. Her weight was dropping into the 170s. Her blood glucose levels had inched down some more. The best news was that her A1C had inched down too, from 8.2% to 7.4%. Both of her clinicians said that was terrific. They complimented her on her hard work taking care of her diabetes.

8

The Food Label Has the Facts

Today supermarkets are nutrient data warehouses! Why? Because of the Nutrition Facts label on most foods. The Nutrition Facts label is front and center because of the revolutionary changes in the food labeling law that went into effect in 1994. These laws were written and are enforced by the U.S. Food and Drug Administration (FDA) and U.S. Department of Agriculture (USDA). The Nutrition Facts label is one of the most complete and up-to-date sources for the nutrient content of foods. And it's free! There's no charge for reading the fine print or for comparing the numbers on several different labels.

As a Carb Counter, you'll find that the listing for Total Carbohydrate in the Nutrition Facts is worth its weight in gold. It's helpful as you learn the carbohydrate content of the foods you eat and when you want to choose new foods.

WHAT FOODS DO NOT HAVE A NUTRITION FACTS LABEL?

Almost all packaged and processed foods have Nutrition Facts labels, but most fresh foods, such as fruits, vegetables, fresh meat, poultry, and fish, do not have the Nutrition Facts label.

Nutrition Facts

Serving Size 1 cup (58g)
Servings Per Container about 8

Amount Per Serving	Multi-Bran Chex	with 1/2 cup skim milk
Calories	200	240
Calories from Fat	15	15
	% Daily Value**	
Total Fat 1.5g*	**2%**	**3%**
Saturated Fat 0g	**0%**	**0%**
Polyunsaturated Fat 0.5g		
Monounsaturated Fat 0g		
Cholesterol 0mg	**0%**	**1%**
Sodium 380mg	**16%**	**19%**
Potassium 220mg	**6%**	**12%**
Total Carbohydrate 49g	**16%**	**18%**
Dietary Fiber 8g	**30%**	**30%**
Sugars 12g		
Other Carbohydrate 29g		
Protein 4g		

WHAT'S ON THE NUTRITION FACTS LABEL?

To get you better acquainted with the Nutrition Facts panel information, let's look at a label from a box of whole-grain dry cereal and break down all of the information it provides.

Nutrition Facts

Nutrition Facts is the title of the list of information about the food. Manufacturers are required by law to provide this information and present it in this same easy-to-read format. The information under the Nutrition Facts heading tells you the Serving Size, the Servings Per Container, Calories, Calories from Fat, Total Fat, Saturated Fat, Sodium, Total Carbohydrate, Dietary Fiber, Sugars, Protein, Vitamins, and Minerals for one serving of the food.

Serving Size. All the nutrition information on the label is based on one serving, **not the whole package** or container. The 1994 law created several improvements to make this information more valuable:

1. Serving sizes are now uniform because the FDA established servings for 139 categories of foods, and manufacturers must use those servings.
2. So-called "reference amounts" are based on the amount of the food that people usually eat.
3. Serving size must be listed in both common household (for example, 4 crackers or 3/4 cup of pasta noodles) as well as metric measures (for example, 28 grams).

Servings Per Container. This is the number of servings in the container.

Calories. This is the number of calories in one serving, listed in bold print.

Calories from Fat. Manufacturers get this number from multiplying the number of grams (g) of fat by 9, because there are 9 calories in 1 g of fat.

Total Fat. The total grams of fat in the serving are listed in bold print.

Saturated Fat. The grams of saturated fat are listed under Total Fat, indented and not in bold print. Saturated fat is part of the total fat. The saturated fat is the only type of fat that must be listed on the label.

Polyunsaturated Fat and Monounsaturated Fat. These are listed under Total Fat, indented and not in bold print. These types of fat are listed voluntarily or if the manufacturer makes a nutrition claim about them.

Trans Fat. Due to the concern about trans fat and heart disease, the FDA, in August of 2003, made the first change to the Nutrition

Facts since their inception nearly a decade prior. Thus, by January 2006 food manufacturers will be required to include on the Nutrition Facts label the number of grams of trans fats in their products.

Cholesterol. The milligrams of cholesterol are listed per serving in bold print.

Sodium. The milligrams of sodium are listed per serving in bold print.

Total Carbohydrate. All the grams of carbohydrate in one serving are listed in bold print. This is the number that you should review when you count carbs. Below Total Carbs and indented in lighter print is Dietary Fiber and Sugars. Sometimes you'll see other sources of carbohydrate or the types of fiber listed. Because sugars, fiber, and other carbohydrates are already counted into the Total Carbohydrate, there is no need to pay special addition to these. More about sugars on page 103. More about how to count fiber below.

Dietary Fiber. The grams of dietary fiber per serving are listed under Total Carbohydrate and indented because fiber is part of the total carbohydrate. There are different types of fiber in foods, and all are considered carbohydrate. Insoluble fibers can't be digested, so they can't be turned into glucose for energy or raise blood glucose levels. Soluble fibers are digested, but at a delayed pace. Some food manufacturers do list the amount of soluble or insoluble fiber in a product if they have something to brag about or if they are required because they have made a nutrition claim about the product's fiber content. The box "Fiber Claims on the Food Label" defines the FDA-allowed fiber claims.

If there are more than 5 g of fiber in the serving of a food that you eat or a meal, *subtract the number of grams of fiber from the grams of total carbohydrate.* Use that number for the carb count in the food. You are subtracting out the grams from fiber since these grams will not raise your blood glucose.

FIBER CLAIMS ON THE FOOD LABEL

Fiber Term	Means
High or excellent source	5 grams or more of fiber per serving
Good source	2.5–4.9 grams per serving
More, enriched, or added	At least 2.5 grams per serving

Sugars. The grams of sugars per serving are listed under Total Carbohydrate and indented because sugars are part of the carbohydrate in the food. Many people with diabetes zero right in on the sugars. There is no need to do this! When you read the Nutrition Facts, look at the grams of Total Carbohydrate *only*. You don't need to single out the grams of sugars. When you count the carbohydrates, you have already counted the sugars.

Protein. The grams of protein per serving are in bold print.

Vitamins and Minerals. Unlike the other information on the Nutrition Facts label, Vitamins and Minerals are not presented as a straightforward measured quantity (like, for example, 8 g of fat). Instead, they are presented as percentages of a Recommended Daily Intake (RDI). There are different RDI levels for certain vitamins and minerals. The food label must list the percentage of the RDI for two vitamins—A and C—and two minerals—calcium and iron. Other vitamins and minerals are listed if the manufacturer makes claims about them. They can also be listed voluntarily. For example, if a food is fortified with folic acid, the Nutrition Facts must state the amount of folic acid per serving.

The Nutrition Facts label does not make it easy to interpret the amount of vitamins or minerals in foods. Most people don't know the RDI amounts for vitamins and minerals. Without these numbers in hand, it is difficult to make any sense out of the information on the label. Table 8-1 gives the RDIs and may help you understand these percentages and make sense of claims on the label. For example, if you look at the label of fat-free milk, you see that a serving has 30% of the RDI for calcium. If you know that the RDI for calcium is 1000 mg, then you can multiply 1000 by .30 to discover that the milk has about 300 mg per 8-oz serving.

Here's another tip. If a manufacturer uses the terms "excellent source of," "rich in," or "high in," the product must contain at least 20% of the RDI for the vitamin or mineral named. If a manufacturer uses the terms "good source of," "contains," or "provides," the product must contain between 10 and 19% of the RDI for that vitamin or mineral. Table 8-1 also provides the amounts of the vitamins and minerals that must be present in a food before "excellent source of" or "good source of" claims can be made.

More about Sugars

It is important to understand that the word "sugars" on the Nutrition Facts panel can only, by FDA definition, be from one-unit sugars—glucose, fructose, galactose—or two-unit sugars—lactose, sucrose, or maltose. These sugars can be:

- Natural sugars, such as the lactose in milk or the sucrose in fruit

- Added sugars, such as corn sweeteners, high-fructose corn syrup, fruit juice, molasses, and brown sugar

Because sugars in foods are from both natural and added sources, there is no way to tell by looking at the grams of sugars on the Nutrition Facts whether the sources are naturally occurring or added. Check for sources of added sugars on the ingredient list. If the added sugars start to stack up, it tells you something about how nutritious—or not—the food is. Perhaps it's best left on the shelf.

T A B L E   8 - 1   The Daily Values and Label Claims for Vitamins and Minerals

Nutrient	Daily value	Excellent source of, rich in, high (20% or greater)	Good source of, contains, provides (10% to 19%)
Potassium	3500 mg	700 mg	350–665 mg
Dietary fiber	25/2000 cal	5 g	2.5–5 g
Vitamin A	5000 IU	1000 IU	500–950 IU
Vitamin C	90 mg (75 mg)	12 mg	6–11 mg
Calcium*	1000 mg	200 mg	100–190 mg
Iron	18 mg	3.6 mg	1.8–3.4 mg
Vitamin D	400 IU	80 IU	40–76 IU
Vitamin E	15 IU (12 IU)	6 IU	3–5.7 IU
Thiamin	1.5 mg	0.3 mg	0.15–0.29 mg
Riboflavin	1.7 mg	0.34 mg	0.17–0.32 mg
Niacin	20 mg	4 mg	2–3.8 mg
Vitamin B6	2 mg	0.4 mg	0.2–0.38 mg
Folate	400 mcg	80 mcg	40–76 mcg
Vitamin B12	6.0 mcg	1.2 mcg	0.6–1.14 mcg
Biotin	0.3 mg	0.06 mg	0.03–0.057 mg
Pantothenic acid	10 mg	2 mg	1–1.9 mg
Phosphorus	1000 mg	200 mg	100–190 mg
Iodine	150 mcg	30 mcg	15–29 mg
Magnesium	400 mg	80 mg	40–76 mg
Zinc	15 mg	3 mg	1.5–2.9 mg
Copper	2.0 mg	0.4 mg	0.2–0.38 mg

*Note:
Calcium: Adults over 51 have a calcium goal of 1200 mg/day.

Sugar-Free, No-Sugar-Added: What's the Lowdown?

Does this sound familiar to you? You were diagnosed with diabetes. When you got over the initial shock, you thought "no more sugars and sweets." On your first trip to the supermarket you sought out the "sugar-free" or "no-sugar-added" foods. Then you began to learn more about diabetes and you realized that sugar is not forbidden and not all sugar-free foods are created equal. To totally digest this topic, it's important to understand a few concepts and have some guidelines to help you decide whether you want to choose these foods and then, how to fit them into your eating plan.

Foods labeled "sugar-free" or "no-sugar-added" aren't necessarily carbohydrate- or calorie-free. How much or little carb they contain depends on what calorie-containing and/or no-calorie-containing sweeteners, as well as other ingredients, are in the food. You've already learned that by FDA food labeling regulations, "sugars" are defined as "all one- and two-unit sugars," such as high-fructose corn syrup, dextrose, or honey. The calorie-containing sweetening ingredients in some sugar-free foods, such as sorbitol or mannitol, aren't "sugars" by FDA definition, but they contain carbohydrate and calories. The no-calorie-containing ingredients in some sugar-free foods, such as aspartame and sucralose, don't contain calories or carbohydrate. Sugar-free foods may or may not cause a blood glucose rise based on the sweeteners and other ingredients in the food.

Sweeteners Used in Sugar-Free Foods

Polyols, also called sugar alcohols, are one group of ingredients in sugar-free foods. Interestingly, they're not sugar or alcohol. They're carbohydrate-based ingredients that contain, on average, half the calories of sugars (2 calories vs. 4 calories per gram); however, some are as low as 0.2 calories per gram and others are as high as 3 calories per gram. Polyols can replace sugar in foods such as candy, cookies, snack bars, and ice creams. Common names are sorbitol, lactitol, maltitol, and mannitol. Note the common "ol" ending.

Polyols contain about half the calories of sugar because they aren't completely digested. Thus, they can cause a lower rise in blood glucose than regularly sweetened foods. However, the calories and grams of carbohydrate per serving of sugar-free foods sweetened with polyols often are only minimally reduced. Observe the comparison of two types of ice creams in Table 8-2. You note that the grams of carb in the no-sugar-added ice cream are as high as the regular. In this case, to know how to count this ice cream you need to have more information—the grams of sugar alcohols. Read on to the section "How to Fit in Sugar-Free Foods" for more.

A downside of sugar alcohols is that in large amounts they can cause gas, cramps, and/or diarrhea. Some people, especially children, can be bothered by this side effect. Foods with certain amounts of polyols are required by the FDA to have a label about this possible "laxative effect."

No-Calorie Sweeteners are another group of ingredients in sugar-free foods. As the name implies, these sweeteners are calorie-free. There are currently five nonnutritive sweeteners approved for use by the FDA—acesulfame-potassium, aspartame, neotame, saccharin, and sucralose. These are used in many foods and beverages today, including diet sodas, fruit drinks, syrups, and yogurts. They contain no calories or carbohydrate and can greatly lower the carbohydrates and calories. They don't, on their own, cause a rise in blood glucose levels.

A Blend of Sweeteners are often used as well. Because there are more polyols and no-calorie sweeteners available to food manufacturers today more combinations of these ingredients are in

T A B L E 8 - 2   Food Labels from Two Ice Creams

Example*

Nutrition Facts
Regular Ice Cream
Serving Size: 1/2 cup

Calories 140	
Total Fat 8g	
Total Carbohydrate 15g	
Sugars 15g	

Nutrition Facts
No-Sugar-Added Light Ice Cream
Serving Size: 1/2 cup

Calories 100	
Total Fat 5g	
Total Carbohydrate 15g	
Sugars 4g	
Sugar Alcohols 3g	

*Shortened label. Not super premium high-fat ice cream.

sugar-free foods. Read ingredient lists to find out what sweeteners are used. By law the ingredient list must tell you.

How to Fit In Sugar-Free Foods

With the ingredient list and the Nutrition Facts label in hand, use Table 8-3 to check out how to fit sugar-free foods into your eating plan.

USE THESE GUIDELINES WHEN ONE OR MORE OF THE INGREDIENTS IN THE FOOD IS A POLYOL:

1. If all the carbohydrate in the food is from polyols and/or no-calorie sweeteners and the Total Carbohydrate is less than 10 g, consider it a "free food." Limit servings to three or less per day.

2. If all the carbohydrate in the food is from polyols and the grams of polyols are greater than 10, then subtract 1/2 the grams of polyols from the Total Carbohydrate grams. Count the remaining carbohydrate grams into your eating plan using Table 8-3.

Nutrition Facts

Sugar-free Hard Candy

(sweetened with malititol and sorbitol)

Serving Size 10 pieces

Calories 80

Total Carbohydrate 36g

  Sugars Alcohols 31g

Example:

31 g of polyols ÷ 2 (half) = 16

36 g of Total Carbohydrate − 16 (1/2 g of polyols) = 20 g of carbohydrate to count. Count as 20 g of carbohydrate or 1 carbohydrate choice.

3. If there are several sources of carbohydrate in the food including polyols, then subtract 1/2 the grams of polyols from the Total Carbohydrate grams. Count the remaining grams of carbohydrate into your eating plan using the chart.

Nutrition Facts

No-Sugar-Added Chocolate Bar

(sweetened with one polyol)

Serving Size: 3 sections (36 g)

Calories 170

Total Carbohydrate 21g

Sugars 3g

Maltitol 16g

Example:

16 g polyols ÷ 2 (half) = 8

21 g of Total Carbohydrate − 8 (1/2 g of polyols) = 13 g of carbohydrate to count. Count as 13 g of carbohydrate or 1 carbohydrate choice.

TABLE 8-3 Fitting in Sugar-Free Foods	
If the food contains a Total Carbohydrate count of:	**Count as:**
0–5 g	A free food
6–10 g	1/2 carbohydrate serving; 1/2 starch, fruit, or milk; or the number of grams of carbohydrate
11–20 g	1 carbohydrate serving; 1 starch, fruit, or milk; or the number of grams of carbohydrate
21–25 g	1 1/2 carbohydrate serving; 1 1/2 starch, fruit, or milk; or number of grams of carbohydrate
26–35 g	2 carbohydrate servings; 2 starch, fruit, or milk; or number of grams of carbohydrate

Sugar-Free Foods: You Be the Judge

Whether you use sugar-free foods and which foods you use is up to you. Now you know more about the ingredients in these foods and how to fit these foods into your eating plan. There is no doubt that many sugar-free foods, especially those sweetened with no-calorie sweeteners, such as diet carbonated and non-carbonated drinks, hot cocoa, yogurt, and syrups, can help quench your sweet tooth without expanding your waistline.

Net Carb, Impact Carb—New Label Lingo

The use of these un-FDA–approved terms started during the low-carb mania brought about by the Atkins diet and other low- or no-carb meal plans. Food manufacturers are using these terms to promote their products to people watching their carb intake and blood glucose levels. To arrive at "net carbs" the manufacturers appear to subtract the total grams of sugar alcohols and fiber from the grams of Total Carbohydrate in the product. The remaining or zero grams of carbohydrate are then referred to as "net carbs." The wording encourages you to count only these grams of carbohydrate as they are the only ones, as stated, to have an impact on blood glucose. Note, the terms and wording varies from label to label.

As part of this new calculation manufacturers provide a statement, which is not necessarily correct, to indicate that only the net carbs in the product have an impact on blood glucose. They do not make any statement about calories. Thus, these new terms are a concern for people with diabetes, especially those who use insulin. Clearly for people who do Advanced Carb Counting and take rapid-acting insulin to cover carbs using the "net carb" information versus the guidelines provided above could cause a person to underestimate his or her insulin need. This could lead to a higher blood glucose level several hours later, without an understandable explanation. Until further notice, it makes the most sense to continue to count polyols as noted above.

It is important to note that the "net carb" information appears outside of the Nutrition Facts panel and to date there are no FDA statements or regulations that have changed the existing definitions of Total Carbohydrate, Sugars, and Sugar Alcohols. However, neither the FDA or USDA seems to be stopping the use of these terms, though they claim that they will define these terms in the near future.

Other Nutrition Claims

Food manufacturers can make other claims on the food label outside of the Nutrition Facts label, such as that the food is calorie free or sugar free. But what do these claims mean? There are guidelines for these claims set up by the food-labeling laws. For an explanation of what they mean, see Table 8-4.

TABLE 8-4 Nutrition Claims on the Food Label	
Nutrition claim	**Means**
Calorie free	Less than 5 calories per serving
Fat free	Less than 0.5 g fat per serving
Sugar free	Less than 0.5 g sugars per serving
Reduced calorie	At least 25% fewer calories than regular food
Reduced fat	At least 25% less fat than regular food
Reduced sugars	At least 25% less sugar than regular food
No added sugar, without added sugar, no sugar added	Permitted if no amount of sugars or ingredient that substitutes for sugar is used, contains no fruit juice concentrate or jelly, and the label says the food is not low calorie

Try Your Hand at Using Food Labels

It will be important for you to be able to use the Nutrition Facts label to do Carb Counting. Use these samples for practice.

1. I often eat cooked oat bran cereal for breakfast. The Nutrition Facts say 1 serving is 1/3 cup and 1 serving contains 19 g of carbohydrate and 5 g of fiber. I eat 2/3 cup as a serving. How many carbohydrate servings are in my serving and do I need to subtract the fiber content? The serving size of 2/3 cup cooked oat bran contains 38 g carbohydrate (19 g + 19 g) and 10 g fiber (5 g + 5 g). You should subtract the grams of fiber because there are more than 5 grams. So 38 g carbohydrate – 10 g fiber = 28 g carb or about 2 carb servings. (Round up to 30 g carb or 2 carb servings.) If you add milk or raisins, or eat other sources of carbohydrate with this breakfast, you will need to add those carbs to your total.

2. For dinner you decide to eat the following foods. You read the Total Carbohydrate on the Nutrition Facts panel for the manicotti, salad dressing, and yogurt. You check the carb count books to get the carb counts for each food that doesn't have a Nutrition Facts label: the roll, salad, and strawberries. Write them down and add it all up.

Item	Carbohydrate (g)
Three-cheese manicotti frozen entrée	41
1 dinner roll	19
1 cup salad greens	–5
2 Tbsp fat-free Catalina dressing	11
1 1/4 cup sliced strawberries	15
1/2 cup orange frozen yogurt	26
Total carbohydrate	117

If you use carbohydrate servings, how many servings would this meal add up to?

117 g carb ÷ 15 = 8 carb servings

3. I often eat dry cereal for a quick breakfast. I mix three cereals together to get a bunch of fiber and the taste I enjoy. I also add 2 Tbsp of raisins. What's the total carbohydrate count for this breakfast?

Item	My cereal (g carb)	Nutrition Facts (g carb)
1/2 cup Bran Flakes	12	24 g in 1 cup (3 g fiber)
1/2 cup Shredded Wheat 'n Bran	23	47 g in 1 cup (5 g fiber)
1/3 cup low-fat Granola	24	48 g in 2/3 cup (2 g fiber)
2 Tbsp raisins	15	15 g in 2 Tbsp (2 g fiber)
1 cup fat-free milk	12	12
Total carb count	86	

My servings of the three cereals are half of the serving sizes listed on the Nutrition Facts panels. I remembered to add the carb count for the raisins and milk, too.

How many carb servings is this breakfast?

86 ÷ 15 = 5 1/2 carb servings

Bonus question #1:
Your cereal breakfast has fiber in it. 3 g + 5 g + 2 g + 2 g = 12 g fiber. What is the carb count of this breakfast?

86 – 12 = 74 g carb

When you subtract the 12 g of fiber from 86, you really are eating 74 grams of carb or 5 carb servings.

Bonus question #2:
How many units of insulin would you need to cover this breakfast if your insulin-to-carb (I:Carb) ratio was 1 to 17?

74 g of carb ÷ 17 units of insulin = 4 units of rapid-acting insulin

9

Convenience Foods and Recipes
HOW TO FIGURE, HOW TO MANAGE

You likely integrate convenience and ready-to-eat foods into the collection of foods you "assemble" into meals during the week for you or your family. Today's convenience and ready-to-eat foods can and do help you put meals together faster and easier. For some of these foods the Nutrition Facts will be in front of your nose and for others you'll need to employ your best "guess-timating" skills.

On the other end of the spectrum, you might enjoy cooking from scratch most of the time or just when the spirit, special occasion, or holiday moves you. You might experiment with a new recipe you clipped from a magazine or new cookbook or use an old family favorite recipe. Unfortunately, there's no carb info on these recipes. Though it will be more difficult to get the carb count, we'll show you in this chapter a process to do just that.

You'll discover that whatever types of foods you eat and ways that you prepare, assemble, or simply heat up meals, you can learn how to fit these foods in with Carb Counting. Your eating style does not have to change because you want to use Carb Counting. In fact, when you become skilled at Carb Counting, you may enjoy using convenience foods or some of your old recipes more because you have the tools you need to take the uncertainty out of what your meals will do to your blood glucose level.

Convenience and Ready-to-Eat Foods

It has been said that today we do more assembling of meals than cooking meals from scratch. Convenience foods are anything from a frozen pizza to a box of macaroni and cheese to a lean frozen entrée. You purchase most of these in the supermarket. When you Carb Count, these convenience foods are actually a blessing because they give you the carb count right on the Nutrition Facts panel.

However, a lot of other convenience or ready-to-eat foods are available these days from a variety of places, such as supermarket deli counters, small independent take-out shops, or large national restaurant chains, such as Boston Market or the many pizza chains. The reality is that today we have an overlap of what's available in supermarkets and some types of restaurants. Nutrition Facts will be available for some of these foods and not for others. For example, at the deli counter, you might be able to ask to see the large container of potato salad to check out the carb count. You'll have the most difficulty obtaining nutrition information for foods prepared in small take-out shops. They don't have to provide nutrition information. That's where your guess-timating skills will come in handy. Regarding restaurants like Boston Market, Pizza Hut, and the like, read chapter 10 to learn more about what information is and isn't available from restaurants and how to access it.

The How To's

Let's start with some frozen convenience foods you might buy in the supermarket. How about frozen pizza? If you are like many Americans, there might be one of these in your freezer at the ready for a quick meal. Here's the Nutrition Facts for a frozen cheese pizza:

Nutrition Facts

Serving Size 1/3 pizza (120 g)

Servings per Container 3

Amount per Serving

Calories 320

Total Fat 13g

  Saturated Fat 6g

Cholesterol 30mg

Sodium 870mg

Total Carbohydrate 35g

  Dietary Fiber 2g

  Sugars 7g

Protein 14g

So, if you eat one serving—or 1/3 of the pizza—it's 35 grams (g) of carb or about 2 carb servings. If you eat one half of the pizza, what would the carb count be?

- If the whole pizza (35 g of carb × 3) contains 105 g of carb, then 1/2 of the pizza contains 53 g of carb or 3 1/2 carb servings.

How about a frozen lean entrée? Here's the nutrition information for a Salisbury Steak with Mashed Potatoes and Green Beans:

Nutrition Facts

Serving Size 1 (269 g)

Servings per Container 1

Amount per Serving

Calories 260

Total Fat 9g

Saturated Fat 4.5g

Cholesterol 45g

Sodium 660mg

Total Carbohydrate 24g

Dietary Fiber 3g

Sugars 4g

Protein 24g

So, the complete entrée is 24 g of carb or about 1 1/2 carb servings. You might add a salad, cup of soup, and/or a dinner roll. Add it all up and you've got your carb count.

How about a canned soup? Here's Lentil Soup with Vegetables:

Nutrition Facts

Serving Size 1 cup (250 g)

Servings per Container about 3

Amount per Serving

Calories 170

Total Fat 1.5g

Saturated Fat 0g

Cholesterol 0g

Sodium 710mg

Total Carbohydrate 30g

Dietary Fiber 7g

Sugars 2g

Protein 10g

So, if you have one cup of soup—or 1/3 of the can—it's 30 g of carb or about 2 carb servings. However, there's one more step on this food. It has 7 g of fiber per serving. Because it's more than 5 g of fiber per serving, you should subtract that amount of fiber from 30 g (30 − 7 = 23 g). So your new total is 23 g of carb or 1 1/2 carb servings. Next, add up the carb from the other items in your meal for your total carb count.

True, these examples are easy because you have the nutrition information right in front of you. Just be sure that you calculate the carbohydrate based on the amount of carb you *actually* eat and not the carb you're *supposed* to eat.

Let's get tougher. You've gotten in the habit of getting a bagel with cream cheese or a muffin at the coffee shop near your office on your way to work each morning. You look at the carb count for a bagel and muffin in Appendix 1. You note that half of a 1-ounce (oz) bagel has 15 g of carbohydrate. You know the bagel you buy is a large bagel. You look up the carb count for a muffin as well. It talks about a 1.5-oz muffin, which contains 15 g of carb. You know the muffin you eat is a "mega" muffin. It just so happens the ones you buy are packaged and list the weight as 6 oz.

So, how do you find nutrition information for these types of foods? You have a couple of choices. One, on a supermarket trip you can see if you find any bagels or muffins that are the size of the ones you get. If they are packaged they will have a Nutrition Facts label. If they are in the bakery they should also have nutrition information. Check out the weight of these bagels and muffins. Eye how close or far they are from the ones you purchase. Then estimate from there. A second approach is to use one of the references in Appendix 2 under Restaurant Foods. Look up bagels and muffin and take an average of the amount of carb in a restaurant or bagel shop bagel. Or use the information gained from both sources and figure it out from there. With all this information—and of course your utmost honesty—you'll likely be very close. Then record the information in your database (see chapter 5), so you don't have to go through this arduous process again.

Here's the nutrition information for a bagel found packaged in the supermarket:

Nutrition Facts

Serving Size 1 (103 g)

Servings per Container 6

Amount per Serving

Calories 264

Total Fat 1.5g

  Saturated Fat 0g

Cholesterol 0g

Sodium 427mg

Total Carbohydrate 53g

  Dietary Fiber 2g

  Sugars 10g

Protein 11g

So, from this information you know this bagel is about 3 1/2 oz (103 g ÷ 30 g in an ounce = 3.5). It contains 53 g of carb or 3 1/2 carb servings. You eyeball it and determine that it's a bit smaller than the one you purchase. Next you check out bagels on the Dunkin' Donuts web site (*www.dunkindonuts.com*). You note that one plain bagel is more like the size of the bagel you buy. There is no weight on it, but you observe the nutrition information.

Nutrition Facts

Serving Size 1

Amount per Serving

Calories 260

Total Fat 3g

  Saturated Fat 0.5g

Cholesterol 0g

Sodium 780mg

Total Carbohydrate 69g

  Dietary Fiber 2g

  Sugars 6g

Protein 14g

You note that this bagel contains 69 g of carbohydrate or 4 1/2 carb servings. You realize you've been topping your carb allotment at breakfast with an innocent bagel. Now, to factor in the cream cheese. You note that one packet of cream cheese only adds 3 g of carb. It does, however, add another 130 calories!

Interestingly, as you go through this process you might actually find that you eat more carb and calories than you thought you were—yes, a rude awakening. If you are trying to lose weight, you might consider making some changes in your food choices. For example, now that you realize the bagel you've been eating contains about 65 g of carb and the bran or corn muffin tops nearly 75 g of carb, you might consider splitting one of either in half and complement it with a piece of fruit to get closer to your carb range for breakfast.

Next, for a couple of quick side dishes for those rushed middle of the week dinners, you regularly stop by the deli counter of the supermarket and buy coleslaw, which is the light vinegar-based type. You also pick up some baked beans—a family favorite. You wonder about their carb counts. One day when the crowd isn't six deep you ask the person behind the counter if you can look at the Nutrition Facts for both items.

You find that the Nutrition Facts on the coleslaw are:

Nutrition Facts
Serving Size 1/2 cup

Amount per Serving

Calories 41

Total Fat 1.5g

   Saturated Fat 0g

Cholesterol 0g

Sodium 14mg

Total Carbohydrate 8g

   Dietary Fiber 1g

   Sugars 3g

Protein 1g

A pleasant surprise. It turns out this coleslaw is an easy way to eat an extra vegetable serving or two without many calories.

You find that the Nutrition Facts for the Barbecued Baked Beans are:

Nutrition Facts

Serving Size 1/2 cup

Amount per Serving

Calories 180

Total Fat 4g

  Saturated Fat 1g

Cholesterol 0g

Sodium 360mg

Total Carbohydrate 32g

  Dietary Fiber 8g

  Sugars 14g

Protein 5g

You know when you eat these you eat much closer to a 3/4 cup serving, so you are probably getting about 48 g of carb. However, there's a good bit of fiber in these beans. At 3/4 cup that's 12 g of fiber that needs to be subtracted from the 48 g of carb. So, that's a grand total of 36 g of carb for the beans.

Again, you add all this new information to your database. No need to go through that exercise every time you eat these foods.

The toughest challenge to counting the carb in ready-to-eat foods will be the foods from a small independent take-out shop that doesn't have nutrition information. That doesn't mean you need to ax these places from your list of options. You have a few methods available. First, ask if they have nutrition information for any of the foods they serve. For example, they might serve a dinner roll that comes in a bag or package that has Nutrition Facts. Second, see if they are willing to let you see a couple of their recipes for dishes that you order all the time. Maybe it's a meat loaf or a chicken stew. Let them know you just need to determine the carb count of a serving. Take a copy of the recipe and do an analysis (you'll learn how in just a bit). Third, you can apply your great guess-timating skills. By now, you are getting pretty good at estimating portions and from there, estimating carb counts. And don't forget, since you are taking the meal home, you do have the opportunity to weigh the portion at home. Check out how much rice or mashed potatoes are on the plate by putting them in a measuring cup.

Meet George

George ate quite a few packaged foods every day, such as frozen pizza, frozen waffles, and boxed macaroni and cheese. He was a very bright young man but always in a hurry. His work schedule had changed, so he was eating breakfast at the early hour of 6 A.M. and lunch was not until 11:30. Around 9 A.M., he was eating a cookie from the vending machine. It was called a Monster Cookie, and he checked the Total Carbohydrate on the food label. It was 35 g. When he checked his blood glucose before lunch or two hours after eating the cookie, it was in the 220–250 mg/dl range. This happened three days in a row. He didn't know why his blood glucose was running high, so he called his dietitian. He had faxed her a copy of the label. She checked the serving size and it was 1 cookie. There were two cookies in the package, and he was eating them both. His morning snack contained 70 g of carbohydrate. Then he realized that he had not been checking the serving size and the number of servings per package. These numbers are as important as the number of grams of carbohydrate. He and his dietitian discussed a plan for better control: eat more breakfast and decrease his morning insulin to prevent low blood glucose mid-morning and eliminate the need for the cookie snack, or find some healthier snacks.

Your Recipes—Counting Carbs

Don't discard your favorite recipes or think that your days of clipping recipes from the newspaper or a magazine are over. Below we show you how to calculate the carb count per serving of recipes.

Certainly one way to avoid this somewhat painstaking exercise is to use recipe books that provide the nutrition information. Obviously what's important to you is the carb count. Note that all of the American Diabetes Association's (ADA) cookbooks provide this information. In addition, most of the cookbooks published that are geared to diabetes, weight loss, and healthier eating also provide carb counts. This is a good way to get new recipes as well as lower-calorie and lower-fat cooking techniques. You can also use these recipes to learn more about the carb counts of certain recipes. All this knowledge is helpful as you learn Carb Counting. There are three cookbooks specifically aimed at Carb Counters:

- *Carb Counting Cookbook*, by Patti Geil, RD, CDE, and Tami Ross, RD, CDE. Wiley and Sons, 1998.

- *Carb Counters Diabetic Cookbook*, by Better Homes and Gardens. Better Homes and Gardens Books, 2003.

- *Quick & Easy Low-Carb Cooking*, by Nancy S. Hughes. American Diabetes Association, 2003.

The How-To's of Recipe Carb Counting

Step #1: Start by writing down each of the ingredients in the recipe and the amount used in the recipe.

Step #2: Then find the grams of carbohydrate that are in the amount of each food in the recipe. The list of foods in Appendix 1 will start you off, then one of the references in Appendix 2 will also be a must. (If you want to know the nutrition information for the other nutrients, such as fat, cholesterol, etc., obtain this information at the same time.)

Step #3: Add up the total grams of carbohydrate from all ingredients in the whole recipe.

Step #4: Divide the total carb by the number of servings to calculate the grams of carbohydrate in one serving.

Step #5: Write this information down on the recipe and/or if it is a recipe you make regularly, write it down in your database of carb counts.

Practice with a Recipe

Find the grams of carbohydrate in this recipe for Morroccan Chicken Stew.

Amount/Ingredients	**Carb (g)**
2 cups chicken broth	0
1/4 cup tomato paste	6
1 tsp ground cumin	0
1 tsp salt	0
1/4 tsp ground red pepper	0
1/8 tsp cinnamon	0
1/2 cup dark raisins	58
1 medium-size onion, sliced thin	16
1 Tbsp minced fresh garlic	4
2 lb butternut squash	52
2 cups frozen green peas	40
1 can (16 oz) chick peas	108
4 chicken thighs	0
Total grams of carbohydrate	**284**

There are 4 servings. Each serving contains 71 g of carb or about 5 carb servings.

As with anything else, practice will increase your comfort level with this process. Select another one of your favorites and take it apart to calculate the grams of carbohydrate.

A Week of Meals from the ADA's *Month of Meals* Series

The following is a week's worth of meals designed to provide the same amount of carbohydrate at each sitting. The *Month of Meals* series, which these meals are borrowed from, is perfect for anyone using Basic Carb Counting or looking to simplify their meal planning with healthy, easy-to-fix recipes. Each book in the series provides twenty-eight days worth of recipes in a split-page format that allows you to make nearly endless combinations of breakfast, lunch, and dinner. No matter what combination you put together, the carb, fat, and calorie counts will fall within your target ranges for the day. This takes so much of the legwork out of Carb Counting, and we highly recommend this series for anyone trying to learn Carb Counting.

The following meal plans should give you an idea of what foods fit into a healthy carb target range for a day, as well as illustrate the breadth and variety of recipes available in the *Month of Meals* series.

MONTH OF MEALS: ALL-AMERICAN FARE

DAY ONE

Breakfast (B): Spanish Omelet, 2 slices rye toast, 1 teaspoon (tsp) margarine, 1/3 cup grapefruit sections

Lunch (L): 1 submarine sandwich, 1/2 large pear, 3 mixed nuts

Dinner (D): 3 ounce (oz) broiled ham with 2 pineapple slices, 2/3 cup cooked brown rice , 1/2 cup steamed carrots with 1 tsp margarine, tossed salad with 2 tablespoon (Tbsp) reduced-fat salad dressing

MONTH OF MEALS: CLASSIC COOKING

DAY TWO

B: 1/2 cup shredded wheat with 1 cup fat-free milk, 1 slice raisin toast with 1 Tbsp cream cheese, 1 sliced peach

L: 1 cup vegetable soup, 1/2 chicken sandwich (1 slice whole-wheat bread, 2 oz chicken breast, 1 tsp mayo, lettuce, tomato, mustard), 1 orange or 1/3 cup frozen fat-free yogurt

D: 1 serving New England Beef Broil,1 slice whole-wheat bread, 1/2 cup cooked spinach, raw celery stix, 3/4 cup raw pineapple cubes or 3 gingersnaps

DAY THREE

B: 1 apple raisin muffin, 1/2 cup bran flakes with 1 cup fat-free milk

L: Chefs Salad, 2 rye krisps, 1 1/4 cup strawberries, 3 oz frozen yogurt

D : 1/2 breast portion of oven-fried chicken, 1 cup mashed potatoes, 2 Tbsp prepared gravy, 1 cup steamed green beans, 1/2 baked apple

MONTH OF MEALS: FESTIVE LATIN FLAVOR (MES DE COMIDAS: SABOR FESTIVO LATINO)

DAY FOUR

B: Breakfast Wrap

L: 1 porcion pescado estilo veracruz

D: 3 oz lomo, vacuno apparrillado, 1 taza ensalada de nopalitos, 2 tortillas, 1 taza papaya

MONTH OF MEALS: SOUL FOOD SELECTIONS

DAY FIVE

B: 1/2 cup grits, 1 poached egg, 1 baked reduced-fat refrigerator biscuit, 1/2 cup orange juice

L: 1 serving Chicken Gumbo Soup, 1 cup mixed vegetables, 2 Tbsp reduced-fat salad dressing, 1 small apple

D: 1 serving Jamaican Style Roast Beef, 2/3 cup cooked rice, 2 cups tossed salad, 2 Tbsp reduced-fat dressing, 1/8 avocado sliced, 1 cup fresh papaya

DAY SIX

B: 1 oz cooked sausage patty, 1 scrambled egg, rolled in 1 8-inch tortilla, 1/2 cup fresh fruit

L: 2 oz baked ham, 1 serving candied sweet potatoes, 1/2 cup cooked collard greens, 1 cup garden salad, 1 Tbsp reduced-fat dressing, 1/4 cup fruit salad, 2 pecan halves

D: 1 serving pork roast, 1 serving pigeon peas and rice, 2 cups tossed salad, 2 Tbsp reduced-fat dressing, 1/2 slice whole-wheat bread, 1/2 tsp margarine, 1 small apple

MONTH OF MEALS: VEGETARIAN PLEASURES

DAY SEVEN

B: 1 whole-wheat currant scone, 2/3 cup fat-free artificially sweetened yogurt

L: 1 bean burger on 1/2 bun topped with Italian-style tomato sauce and 1 oz part-skim mozzarella cheese slice, 1 tsp margarine, 1/3 oz pretzels, and 1 small nectarine

D: 1 serving spinach lasagna, 1 roll, 2 tsp margarine, 1/2 cup fresh fruit salad

10

Restaurant Meals
HOW TO FIGURE, HOW TO MANAGE

Eating out at restaurants and bringing restaurant foods home or to work has become the way Americans tackle the job of eating. That's because most of us have hectic busy lives, and today restaurant foods are available nearly 24/7. The average American eats four or more restaurant meals each week. Many of you probably top that number. The good news is that if restaurant meals are part of the way you eat, this doesn't have to change with Carb Counting. In fact, when you become skilled at Carb Counting, you may be able to enjoy restaurant meals more and have your blood glucose in better control because you have the tools and the knowledge you need.

Restaurant Foods: Eat In or Take Out

Get a clearer idea of your restaurant eating habits by asking yourself these questions.

1. Which meals and snacks do you eat away from home, during the day, week, or month? Are you more likely to eat out during the day or the evening?
2. Why do you eat meals at a restaurant?
   - Convenience
   - Lack of time

■ To get a variety of foods
■ Not interested in cooking
■ Like to be served
■ Food tastes good

3. What is your typical order in your favorite types of restaurants? What quantities of food do you eat?

Write down what you eat in your favorite restaurants. Estimate the size of the serving and the amount of carbohydrates in it. If you have information on your blood glucose levels after eating out, put that down, too. These records will provide clues about how well you estimate the carbohydrate in your restaurant meals. Also write down the beverages you drink, whether they are carbonated, fruit juices, alcoholic, or calorie free. Some of these beverages have carbohydrates and calories, and you may not realize how much you consume.

Now, do you have a better picture of your restaurant eating style? Your records provide the data you need to count the carb servings or grams of carbohydrate in the foods you eat away from home. Check the food lists in this book or in the resources listed in Appendix 2 to help you count the carbs in your restaurant meals. Also read on in this chapter.

When you eat out, do you follow your meal plan or ignore it? Do you overeat in certain restaurants or at certain times of the day? What can you learn about yourself from your food records? Get the menu from your favorite restaurants and go to the web for the menus of national fast food chains. Make a list of the foods and dishes you order and figure the carb counts before you go to the restaurants again. Add the carb counts for these meals to your database of carb counts. That way you won't have to keep recalculating.

Restaurant Foods—How to Estimate Carb Content

No doubt, when you have nutrition information in hand it makes Carb Counting a snap. That's easy when you have a food package

with the Nutrition Facts label or you look at a web site that over-
flows with nutrition data. But, it's not as easy when you stare down
your entrée at a local family-run restaurant. Counting the carbs of
restaurant foods can be more challenging. The tips below can help
you become an expert restaurant Carb Counter with practice.

RESTAURANT NUTRITION INFORMATION: WHAT IS AND ISN'T AVAILABLE?

Today there's more nutrition information available for restaurant
foods than ever before, but by no means is nutrition information
available for all restaurant foods. Here's the lowdown.

There is nutrition information available from so-called "walk
up and order" national chain restaurants for all the menu items.
That's McDonald's, Domino's, KFC, etc. The best place to access
the information is through their web sites. The nutrition information may also be available at the restaurant in a nutrition facts
brochure or on a poster posted in the restaurant. But, that's a
maybe. Plus, the poster may be in microscopic print posted closer
to the ceiling than at eye level. So, take a few minutes to cruise the
web sites of your favorite "walk up and order" national chain
restaurants. Look for the menu items you tend to order and record
the carb counts in a format similar to Table 10-1 so you'll have
them at your fingertips when you need them.

On the converse, nutrition information is hard to come by for
"sit down and order" type restaurants. That's true for the many
national chains, such as Applebee's, TGI Fridays, and Chili's, as
well as regional and local chains and independent restaurants. The
national chain restaurants claim that it's difficult for them to provide this information because their foods and their preparation
varies from one restaurant to another. Interestingly, however, some
chain restaurants do manage to provide nutrition information for
items they want to promote as healthy or low carb. These are generally few and far between. Some of these chains do suggest that
people contact their corporate customer service office to inquire
about a few items of interest. It's even harder to find nutrition

information for the vast majority of your regional and local chains and independent restaurants. This is understandable because it can be costly to obtain this information. Therefore, your best defense is to have done your homework at home and to follow the "Tips to Make Your Best Guess" section below.

The good news is that just as with foods you eat at home, the same is true with restaurant foods. You generally frequent the same restaurants over and over, and generally you go there because you like and order certain dishes. So, if you are at Mama Leoni's Italian Garden you will order either lasagna or veal cacciatore. If it's Mexican, you will order fajitas or enchiladas. You get the picture. For this reason, it does make sense for you to spend some time estimating the nutrient content of the few restaurant items that you eat for which nutrition information is not available. Then add this information to your database so you have it at your fingertips (example: Table 10-1).

TIPS TO MAKE YOUR BEST GUESS:

- Become familiar with portions of foods. For example, know what a 6-ounce (oz) baked potato, 1 cup of rice, or a 3-oz hamburger look like. The best way to get these visions in your mind is to have, and regularly use, measuring equipment at home. That's back to the principles in chapter 7. If you weigh and measure foods regularly at home you'll get and keep your eyes familiar with portions. This feel will help you closely estimate portions in restaurants. Estimating portions correctly helps you estimate the carb counts correctly.

- Remember you have a "handy" guide (page 94) available to you at all times—your hands. Use these as you try to estimate restaurant portions.

- "Borrow" the scales in the produce aisle of a supermarket to become knowledgeable about the servings of foods you may

TABLE 10-1 **Sample Personal Database Record–Restaurant Meals**

Meal	Serving (amount I eat)	Grams of Carb
Restaurant: Burger King		
Original Whopper Jr. (hold mayo)	1	32
French fries	1/2 medium	23
Side garden salad	1	5
Salad dressing–Catalina	2 Tbsp	5
Total		**65**
Restaurant: Pizza (from local pizza parlor)*		
Cheese with onions and mushrooms pizza	3 slices	96
Total		**96**
Restaurant: Mexican (from local Mexican restaurant)**		
Fajitas with	3	
Chicken and beef	4 oz	0
Grilled onions and peppers	2/3 cup	11
Tortillas–6 in.	3	54
Guacamole	3 Tbsp	4
Tomatoes	1/2 cup	3
Rice–Mexican	1/3 cup	16
Refried beans	1/2 cup	20
Total		**108**

* Estimate based on an average of nutrition information from Pizza Hut, Domino's, and Papa John's from *Guide to Healthy Restaurant Eating*, American Diabetes Association, 2002.
** Based on Nutrition Facts labels and Nutrition Information obtained from *www.nal.usda.gov/fnic/foodcomp/* (the USDA searchable database).

RESTAURANT NUTRITION LABELING LAWS

There is a growing momentum from nutrition and health experts to encourage, or shall we say force, restaurateurs to provide nutrition information. This has been in the form of the introduction of legislation. Bills have been introduced in several state legislatures, such as New York, Maine, California, and the District of Columbia and in both the Federal House of Representatives and the Senate. The House Resolution (HR. 3444) was introduced by Rep. DeLauro (D-CT) in November 2003 and the Senate Bill (S. 2108) was introduced by Sen. Tom Harkin (D-IA) in February 2004. You can view the details of these bills at the web site *http://thomas.loc.gov*. If you are supportive of this type of legislation and want to make your voice heard, contact your state and federal legislators.

---

be served in a restaurant, such as a baked white or sweet potato, an ear of corn, or a banana. Weigh individual pieces of these foods. Check out how many ounces a usual potato or ear of corn is that you may be served in a restaurant. (You weigh these foods raw, but their weight doesn't change that much when they're cooked.)

■ If no nutrition information is available for particular restaurants you frequent, use the information available from other similar restaurants. For example, if you want to get a feel for the nutrient content of a food like French fries, baked potatoes, stuffing, baked beans, pizza, bagels, and others, look at the serving size and nutrition information for those foods served in restaurants for which there is nutrition information on the restaurant's web site or in the nutrition resources noted in Appendix 2. You might want to take a few examples and then do an average. For example, if you regularly eat at a local pizza shop rather than a national chain and they have no nutrition information, get the nutrition information for two slices of a medium-size regular crust cheese pizza from three restaurants. Then do an average. You will come pretty close to the nutrition content of the three slices of cheese pizza you eat (see example in Table 10-1).

- If no nutrition information is available for particular restaurants you frequent, use the Nutrition Facts from similar foods in the supermarket. For example, you might find similar frozen or packaged foods. Consider frozen pizza, macaroni and cheese, spinach soufflé, chicken pot pie, and the like. Again, take a couple of examples and then do an average.

- If you regularly eat particular cultural foods for which you find no nutrition information, you might want to get a few cookbooks out of the library (or use your own) that contain recipes for the foods you enjoy. Then use a nutrient database or book with nutrition information such as those listed in Appendix 2 to determine the estimated nutrient content for each ingredient. This might work well for cultural foods such as Japanese, Chinese, or Thai. You'll learn that the sauces in some of the dishes contain sources of carbohydrate that you can't account for by just looking at the dish in a restaurant. For example, sushi rice contains added sugar and Chinese sauces often contain sugar, sweet sauces, or corn starch. No wonder your blood glucose may rise after you eat these foods.

Restaurant Eating: Tips and Skills

One of the biggest problems with restaurant meals is that the portions are *huge*. Here are tips and tactics to help you control your portions:

- Be on the lookout for the words on the menu that mean large portions—large, giant, grande, supreme, extra large, jumbo, double, triple, double-decker, king-size, and super. Search for the words that mean small portions—junior, single, petite, kiddie, and regular. No surprise, the smaller-portion adjectives are harder to find.

- If you see a weight for a piece of meat on the menu, it's most likely the raw weight. For example, you might see a hamburger referred to as a "quarter pound" of meat or a filet weighing 6 oz, or a slice of prime rib that weighs 10 oz. Remember that these are average—not exact—weights. Apply the rule of thumb on page 97 to help you convert servings from raw weight to cooked weight. Also keep in mind that entrée portions of meat in sit-down restaurants are often enough for two people. (It might be best to split the portions or ask for a take home container when you order.)

- Think about ordering a soup and salad, or appetizer and soup. That may be enough for you. Or see if you can order a half portion. This is particularly easy to do with pasta entrées. Ask whether your dining partner is willing to share. For example, in a steak house, one person orders the steak (which is enough for two) and the other person orders side orders of a baked potato, salad, or vegetable. Consider splitting two entrees that complement each other. For example, in an Italian restaurant, one person orders pasta topped with a tomato-based sauce and the other orders a chicken, veal, or fish dish. Split both dishes and you each have a more balanced meal. Or you can all eat family or "Asian" style— share several dishes among several people. True, we said earlier to stop doing this, but if you order fewer dishes than the number of people at the table (instead of the other way around), this is a good way to cut portions.

- Know when enough is enough. Don't clean your plate. Take the extras home. It's a good idea not to wait until you're stuffed to figure out what the extras are. Ask for a take-home container when you order your meal. Divide the meal and put the half you want for tomorrow's leftovers away before you dig in.

■ You might want to go a step further than just eyeing portions, especially if your blood glucose seems to be hard to control after your favorite restaurant meals. You could order one or two of your favorite items to take home. At home, carefully weigh and measure the portions. See if your eye measurements are accurate or if you greatly under- or overestimated. The next time you order that food in your favorite restaurant, you will be able to adjust your medication more precisely to control your blood glucose levels. Or you may eat more carefully, so you get only the serving you need (see chapter 13).

A Closer Look—Lunch at a Restaurant

When you eat lunch at a restaurant, remember your target range for carbs. Maybe it's 45, 60, or 75 grams (g). Soup and salad are usually considered a light lunch. But, it depends on what you put on your salad and what type of soup you have: one that's broth based or one that's cream based, full of beans, and pasta. Let us take a look at a "light lunch."

Food	Carbohydrate (g)
3 cups salad greens	8
bacon bits, egg, ham	0
1/3 cup kidney beans	15
1/3 cup garbanzo beans	15
1 cup croutons	15
1/3 cup fat-free salad dressing	15
1 1/2 cups chicken noodle soup	30
Total carbohydrate	**98, or 6 1/2 carb choices**

A so-called "light" lunch can easily put you way above even 75 g of carb. How can you get this meal into your target range for carbs?

- Reduce the amount of croutons to 1/2 cup and save 8 g of carb.

- Reduce the salad dressing to 1 Tbsp and save 12 g of carb.

- Combine the kidney and garbanzo beans in a 1/3 cup serving and save 15 g of carb.

- Add 1 cup of a combination of broccoli, cauliflower, and carrots for 5 g of carb.

- Only have 1 cup of the soup and save 10 g of carb.

Your total saving is 45 g of carbohydrate, and you're back in range without giving up too much flavor or quantity of food.

Meet JB | JB ate all his lunches at the food court of the local mall during the workweek. He rotated his choices from the various ethnic cafes at the food court. The selections varied among Greek, Chinese, Japanese, Mexican, and Italian. He had the habit of ordering the same item from each of the places, and he selected each one on a specific day. He was concerned about his blood glucose levels, and he had learned by keeping food and blood glucose records that with some meals he had good glucose levels after the meal and with others his levels were too high. He was trying to eat a certain range of carbohydrate grams. So his dietitian suggested that they do a "food lab" with his food choices. He bought one of each item that he usually ordered, and they measured the carb counts of each. His target for grams of carbohydrates at lunch was 60–75 g. Typically, he orders:

Chinese: vegetable stir-fry with a bowl of fried rice

Mexican: two beef enchiladas (small)

Greek: a gyro sandwich with cucumber salad

Japanese: a plate of sushi with miso soup

Italian: two slices of deep-dish pizza with a small garden salad and Thousand Island dressing

He and his dietitian measured the servings with measuring cups and a food scale to figure the actual amount of carbs in each meal. JB thought all of them contained between 60 and 75 g of carbohydrate.

Chinese. They measured the amount of fried rice in the bowl. It should have been 1 1/2 cups. The actual amount was 2 1/2 cups, which has 105 g of carbohydrate. The stir-fry veggies were all non-starchy vegetables, such as broccoli and bok choy, and there was 1 1/2 cup of them, or 15 g of carb. This meal had 120 g of carb, which was nearly twice as much as the 60–75 g target range. When he checked his blood glucose level after the meal, it was 235 mg/dl. This showed that the larger amount of carbs raised his blood glucose higher than he wanted it to be 2 hours after the meal.

Mexican. His two beef enchiladas had 35 g of carbohydrate—much less than his target level. When he checked his blood glucose level 2 hours later, it was 60 mg/dl, and he had to treat a low blood glucose level (hypoglycemia). He needed to add either a serving of Mexican rice or refried beans to his lunch for more carb in the meal.

Greek. The gyro sandwich had thick pita bread as the wrap, and it was filled with lean lamb. The wrap weighed 2 oz, so it counted as 30 g of carbohydrate. The cucumber salad was 1 cup of cucumbers and 1/3 cup of yogurt, equal to 5 g of carbohydrate. The lamb had no carb, so this was much below his target of 60–75 grams of carbohydrate. They checked his blood glucose log, and it showed a glucose level of 65 mg/dl after the meal. He had low blood glucose. He needed to add a medium-sized piece of fruit and a glass of milk for 30 g of carbohydrate or a total of 62 g of carb in the meal.

Japanese. The rice in the sushi is the source of the carbohydrate in the meal. Fortunately, he really likes sushi, so he eats enough rolls to reach his target of 60 g of carbohydrate.

Italian. He enjoys eating the deep-dish three-cheese pizza. Each large slice of the pizza has 37 g of carbohydrate, and he was eating two large slices. With a total of 74 g of carbohydrate in this lunch, his blood glucose level 2 hours later was 185 mg/dl—higher than he wanted it. He planned to have smaller pieces of the pizza in the future. The dietitian suggested that thin-crust pizza is healthier, especially with only a regular amount of cheese and some veggies, such as mushrooms, peppers, and onions.

Keeping blood glucose records helped them see the effect of the carbohydrate on his blood glucose, so they could make adjustments in what he ate. For the days he ate Mexican or Greek, he needed to add some foods with more grams of carbohydrate. On the days he ate Chinese and Italian, he needed to adjust his servings so they are not so large, and he ate fewer grams of carbohydrate. He found this exercise very useful because he could continue to eat the variety of foods that he enjoyed. But now he knew the amount of carbohydrate in each of the food items, so his blood glucose stayed within healthy ranges.

If you eat at a variety of places and you want an estimated carb count for each entrée, this type of exercise is helpful. You can do a food lab on your own or get the help of your dietitian the first time you try it, and then do it at home as your restaurant choices expand.

11

Blood Glucose Pattern Management
A KEY TO FINE-TUNING YOUR CONTROL

Now you know a lot about what carbs are, what carbs do to your blood glucose levels, and how to count the carb in the wide variety of foods you eat. You also know what your target blood glucose levels should be (see page 7 in chapter 1). What's next? Learning to use the data you record each day—carbs you eat, diabetes medications you take and when, your blood glucose measurements, and more—to help you gain insight into your blood glucose patterns.

This insight and learning will help you and your diabetes health care providers fine-tune your blood glucose control through what diabetes health care providers call "pattern management." Pattern management is simply a way to use your records to learn about your body's reaction to everything you do and then to figure out how to adjust your diabetes plan and your daily activities to get the best blood glucose control you can.

Does this mean you can expect to get to a point in the near future where your blood glucose levels will be in perfect control? Unfortunately for most people with diabetes, that's not the case. But there are two pieces of good news. One, you can minimize the roller coaster ride, moving from the giant roller coaster to the one that doesn't leave your stomach a few feet behind or above you. Two, from research studies it is known that if your blood glucose levels are in your target zones the majority of the time, you can keep yourself healthy—both day to day and for years to come.

No doubt, managing blood glucose levels can be quite frustrating. There are days you do everything just like you did the day before, when all your blood glucose results were perfect, only to find your blood glucose levels completely out of whack. Do you

ADJUST DIABETES MEDICATIONS: WHO?

When you read about adjusting your diabetes medications you may wonder if this applies to you. That's a great question. The answer depends on a few things, such as:

- What diabetes medicines you use to treat your diabetes and if these can be adjusted

- How comfortable you and your diabetes health care provider feel with you making these adjustments

- How much time you are willing and able to take to check your blood glucose regularly and do pattern management

Generally speaking, people with type 2 diabetes who take oral diabetes medications, such as one of the sulfonylureas, metformin or a glitazone—which are the most commonly used today—do not adjust their medications during the day or from day to day. However, if you have type 1 diabetes you will want to do pattern management to collect data on your blood glucose control and share this with your diabetes health care provider to evaluate whether your diabetes plan is keeping you in good control or if not, how to change it to get you into your target ranges.

Generally speaking, people with type 1 diabetes or those people with type 2 diabetes who take at least four insulin injections a day or who use an insulin pump will be able to learn to adjust their insulin doses from meal to meal. It is the rapid-acting insulin that you will adjust most frequently.

throw up your hands in frustration? Yes, sometimes! But keep in mind that Carb Counting and managing blood glucose levels is an art—not a science. It isn't possible to keep blood glucose in perfect control all the time because blood glucose results do not reflect just the carbohydrate in foods. Blood glucose levels depend on what your blood glucose level was before you ate, the stress you're under, your physical activity (yesterday and today), your level of insulin resistance all the time and at different times of the day, how much protein and fat was part of the meal, how fast or slowly you ate, and on and on and on.

Keep in mind, you are a unique individual, and every time you sit down to eat, it is a new physical-chemical-emotional interaction. The only way to get a handle on the many factors that can affect your blood glucose is to build your own "database of experiences." In other words, keep records so you can learn from a wide variety of your personal experiences. Track your individual reactions and responses to different foods and different situations. This data (or feedback) will help you know how your body is likely to react and help you make the adjustments you need to make for the wide variety of situations that life brings along.

LET'S CONSIDER A COUPLE OF EXAMPLES WITH FOOD

Say your favorite dessert is cheesecake. You have a piece at your favorite restaurant a few times a year. The next time you enjoy a wedge, you check your blood glucose one and two hours after and again four to five hours later to see the impact of this dessert on your blood glucose level. So, what does the cheesecake do to your blood glucose? Did you guess right about how much insulin you need to cover the cheesecake (and the rest of the meal)? What did you learn from the experience? What will you do differently the next time? Now jot some notes down in your database of experiences so you'll remember how you want to handle this experience next time.

Next. You enjoy going for long hikes. You take a mixture of raisins and peanuts with you to eat along with a light lunch. You decrease the amount of insulin you take because you know you will burn more calories and lower your blood glucose that way. So what happens? Is this enough food or do you need a second sandwich? Did you decrease your insulin too much because your blood glucose went higher than you thought it might?

Learning from your own experiences and from monitoring the reaction of your blood glucose will help you control your diabetes more than anything else. Eventually, you'll be able to predict how your body will react in most of the usual daily situations.

What Should You Record?

To do pattern management you need to keep records. The records should detail the following information:

- Foods and beverages you consume with their carb counts

- Times of meals and snacks

- Dose, type, and time of diabetes medications (pills or insulin)

- Times of blood glucose check and result

- Types and length of physical activity

- Whether it is a workday, school day, weekend, or other type of day

- Changes such as illness, physical or emotional stress, menstruation

Unfortunately, the small record-keeping logs that come with most of the blood glucose meters don't provide enough room to record this information. They mainly concentrate on your blood glucose results and medications. And we know there's a lot more to the why's and wherefore's of blood glucose levels than this. For a sample recording form, check out Appendix 3. For examples of how these are used, review the later part of this chapter.

Pattern Management—It Takes Three Steps

Here's the three-step process of pattern management.

STEP 1. FIND THE PATTERNS

What do you need?

- A few weeks of blood glucose records that contain at least two blood glucose checks each day

- Two color markers or highlighters—one for high levels (above the targets below), one for low levels (below 70 mg/dl)

- Your blood glucose targets. Talk with your health care providers about your target blood glucose levels. In general, ideal blood glucose target ranges are:

  - Before meals: 90–130 mg/dl (plasma)

  - After meals (one to two hours after start): less than 180 mg/dl (plasma)
    Note: When you use Carb Counting, checking your blood glucose two hours after you start to eat a meal is the only way to see what effect the diabetes medication or activity (or both) has on your blood glucose after eating.

STEP 2. OBSERVE THE PATTERNS

If many of your blood glucose results are *above* your target range, consider whether one or several of the following could be the cause:

- Not taking the correct dose of medication, the dose needs to be increased, or you need additional or different medications

- Too much carbohydrate at the meal

- Less physical activity than planned

- Physical or emotional stress

- A high-protein and/or high-fat meal

If many of your blood glucose values are *below* the target range consider whether one or several of the following could be the cause:

- Delayed or missed meals or snacks

- Too little carbohydrate at meals or snacks

- Diabetes medication taken incorrectly or dose needs adjustment

STEP 3. PLAN AND TAKE ACTION

With your observations in mind, plan your actions to increase the number of blood glucose results that are in your target range. Then take action, if this action is within your comfort zone. For example, you may have found that most evenings a couple hours after dinner your blood glucose is high. You believe the cause of this is that you're eating more carb than you should at dinner. Therefore, a logical action would be to eat the amount of carb you *should* be eating, then check your blood glucose a few evenings to determine if this change has brought your blood glucose levels into your target range. This is an action you're comfortable with and it can bring positive results.

Medication can sometimes be a little different. Changing your dosage may have a positive effect, but many people don't feel comfortable adjusting their medication, which is understandable.

If you don't adjust your medications yourself, then bring your observations with you to your next appointment. If your blood glucose results are consistently dangerously high (above 250 mg/dl) or low (below 70 mg/dl), then don't wait until your next visit with your diabetes health care provider with your observations. Contact them immediately.

Is there Data Management Technology for Pattern Management?

Yes. Today, most of the blood glucose monitors double as a data management system. They record your blood glucose results in the memory. The results are downloadable to your personal computer with the assistance of software provided by or purchased from the company. There is a range of what's available and how to utilize the information. Several meters allow you to record on the meter the type and dose of insulin. One meter (FreeStyle Tracker) is available integrated with a PDA (personal digital assistant). It stores up to 2,500 results, has a food database with carb counts, and has reminder alarms to check blood glucose levels. The data from the PDA can be downloaded to a personal computer. One of the pump companies (Animas Corporation; *www.animascorp.com*) has a data management system, *ez*Manager Plus, that can be downloaded to a Palm Pilot. It contains the carb counts for several thousand foods. It allows you to track insulin doses, activity, and more. Any of these systems can make record keeping and pattern management much easier.

To investigate these, the best advice is to go to the web site of the company whose meter you use. See what data management system and software they have. If you want to find out the breadth of what's available, check out the options listed in Appendix 2 under software for PDAs. Also, each fall the American Diabetes Association's *Diabetes Forecast* publishes their "Resource Guide." It is a terrific resource to learn all about all the diabetes products available, including data management systems.

Time for Real Life Practice

The rest of this chapter contains the sample records of people with type 1 and type 2 diabetes. Then each of the records has been put through the three pattern management steps. Observe how these people have analyzed their records. This will give you hands-on experience with pattern management. These sample logbooks use the record form in Appendix 3. Due to space constraints, it's difficult to provide many days of data and details. A couple of the people have four days of records.

Meet FW

FW is newly diagnosed with type 2 diabetes and does not take diabetes medication yet. He is 45 years old. He is 5'10" tall and weighs 225 pounds. His target blood glucose (BG) range for fasting and before meals is 90–130 mg/dl and for two hours after meals is less than 180 mg/dl. He wanted to give Carb Counting a try, so he kept a log of two meals for a day to see how much carb he was eating and the effect it had on his BG levels. He did not have target carbohydrate goals because he did not know how much he was eating at meals. His record of two meals on one day is on pages 152–153.

STEP 1. FIND THE PATTERNS

FW's records show that he started his day with a high BG level of 240 mg/dl. He had 124 g of carb at breakfast and a BG of 308 mg/dl two hours after breakfast. His BG level before lunch was 228 mg/dl. He had 139 g of carbohydrate at lunch and a BG of 318 mg/dl two hours after lunch. This showed him that his BG levels were way higher than his before- and after-meal targets. He was now understanding why he had symptoms of high blood glucose, such as thirst and having to urinate a lot.

STEP 2. OBSERVE THE PATTERNS

He was able to see a pattern. He started his day with a high BG. His breakfast and lunch carbohydrate grams were in the 124–139 range, which was too high and was causing the high after-meal BG levels. He did no physical activity before or after those meals to help bring the high BG levels down. This information helped him make some decisions.

STEP 3. PLAN AND TAKE ACTION

FW decided to add some physical activity during the day: a 15-minute walk after lunch. He discussed the amount of carbohydrate he should eat at his meals with a dietitian. He said he was willing to cut down some and shoot for a range of 80–90 g of carb per meal. Then he would keep records for three days (a weekend day and two workdays) and go through the three-step process again to see if he needed to make further adjustments.

Meet Roberta

Roberta had learned Carbohydrate Counting and was keeping records to see if she could achieve her target BG goals. She is 60 years old, lives alone, and has type 2 diabetes. She has a target BG goal, fasting and before meals, of 120 mg/dl, and a two-hour after-meal BG target of 190 mg/dl. She takes two diabetes pills, Amaryl and Actos (see her medication record on pages 154–155). She was keeping this record to see how much carbohydrate she was eating, how it affected her BG level, and whether her physical activity and medication had a positive effect on her BG levels.

STEP I. FIND THE PATTERNS

Roberta checked for BG levels that were in or out of range. Her fasting, after breakfast, before lunch, after lunch, before dinner, and after dinner were all out of range.

FW's Carbohydrate Counting and Blood Glucose Results Record

Day/Date: *Monday*

Time/ meal	Diabetes medicines		Food		Carb count (servings/ grams)
	Type	Amount	Type	Amount	
8:30 A.M./ breakfast	None		Sausage	2	0
			Biscuit, 2 oz	1	34
			Banana, med.	1	30
			Orange juice (fast food)	16 oz	60
					Total 124
2:00 P.M. lunch	None		Cheeseburgers, Jr.	2	68
			Fries	small	33
			Chocolate chip cookies (fast food)	3	38
					Total 139

Notes about day:

Roberta's Carbohydrate Counting and Blood Glucose Results Record

Day/Date: *Saturday*

Time/ meal	Diabetes medicines		Food		Carb count (servings/ grams)
	Type	Amount	Type	Amount	
8:00 A.M./ breakfast	Glucovance	500 mg	Oatmeal, 1 pkg	1 cup	68
			Whole milk	1 cup	12
			Banana	1 large	25
					Total 105
12:30 P.M. lunch			Macaroni & cheese	2 cups	54
			Apple juice	1 cup	30
					Total 84
6:30 P.M. dinner	Glucovance	500 mg	Soup–chicken noodle, Campbell's	2 cups	30
			Crackers–saltine	12	12
			Canned mixed fruit cocktail, water packed	1 cup	22
					Total 64

Notes about day:

Blood glucose results

Fasting/ before b'fast/ time	After b'fast/ time	Before lunch/ time	After lunch/ time	Before dinner/ time	After dinner/ time	Before bed/ time	Other/ time
240 (7:35 A.M.)	308 (10:00 A.M.)						
		228 (1:45 P.M.)	318 (3:45 P.M.)				

Blood glucose results

Fasting/ before b'fast/ time	After b'fast/ time	Before lunch/ time	After lunch/ time	Before dinner/ time	After dinner/ time	Before bed/ time	Other/ time
174 (7:30 A.M.)	208 (10:15 A.M.)						
		196 (12:15 P.M.)	280 (1:45 P.M.)				
				180 (6:15 P.M.)	216 (7:50 P.M.)		30-minute walk before dinner

Roberta's Blood Glucose Records

Day/Date (fill in times)	12A	3A	6A	B'4 Meal	2 hr aft. Meal	Other	B'4 Meal	2 hr aft. Meal	Other	B'4 Meal	2 hr aft. Meal	Other
Blood glucose				189	275		170	225		160	218	
Carb grams					88			92			95	

Day/Date (fill in times)	12A	3A	6A	B'4 Meal	2 hr aft. Meal	Other	B'4 Meal	2 hr aft. Meal	Other	B'4 Meal	2 hr aft. Meal	Other
Blood glucose				170	200		155	199		168	211	
Carb grams					75			79			84	

Day/Date (fill in times)	12A	3A	6A	B'4 Meal	2 hr aft. Meal	Other	B'4 Meal	2 hr aft. Meal	Other	B'4 Meal	2 hr aft. Meal	Other
Blood glucose				183	276		173	252		181	266	
Carb grams					77			81			71	

Roberta reviewed her 3 day blood glucose records with the dietitian from her diabetes team over the phone, and she saw a pattern with elevated premeal blood glucose levels, and also higher carb intake than her carb budget would allow. The dietitian recommended she increase her Actos to 45 mg, and try to stay on her carb budget. The dietitian encouraged her to fax in her records next week and to set up a phone call to review them.

Day/Date (fill in times)	12A	3A	6A	B'4 Meal	2 hr aft. Meal	Other	B'4 Meal	2 hr aft. Meal	Other	B'4 Meal	2 hr aft. Meal	Other
Blood glucose				135	177		125	168		135	159	
Carb grams					70			77			70	

Roberta faxed in her records and called in at the time she and her dietitian had set up. Her records indicated that the increase in the Actos and her more careful attention to her carb counts were keeping her blood glucose closer to her targets. She was very encouraged. She planned to continue with this plan as well as her walking program for the next month.

STEP 2. OBSERVE THE PATTERNS

She looked for patterns. She found that she ate too much carb at breakfast. Over 100 g was simply too much. She was delighted to see that a 30-minute walk before dinner helped keep the after-meal BG lower than it was after lunch with the same amount of carbohydrate. However, it was still too high. She also noticed that her fasting BG was high—174 mg/dl.

STEP 3. PLAN AND TAKE ACTION

She decided to cut her breakfast down to 1/2 cup of oatmeal, use low fat milk (which saves calories, but not carbs), and add 1/2 banana. That will cut her carbs to about 75 g. She will also try to eat smaller portions at lunch and dinner and keep that carb count to between 65 and 75 g.

This is a middle step, as these are still high amounts for a small lady like Roberta. She was willing to keep logs for a few days with these changes and see what effect they had on her BG levels. Since Roberta is not taking the maximal dose of either of her diabetes medications and she has had type 2 diabetes for about eight years, it might be that she needs more medication. She will discuss her records and observations with her health care provider at her upcoming visit.

DT's Carbohydrate Counting and Blood Glucose Results Record

Day/Date: *Tuesday*

Time/meal	Diabetes medicines		Food		Carb count (servings/grams)
	Type	**Amount**	**Type**	**Amount**	
8:30 A.M./ breakfast	Lispro	5 units	Skim milk	1 cup	12
			Raisin toast	2	26
			Margarine	1	0
					Total 38
2:00 P.M. lunch	Lispro	5 units	Tuna (sandwich)	3 oz	0
			Bread	2 slices	30
			Mayonnaise	1 Tbsp	0
			Apple–large	1	30
					Total 60
5:30 P.M. dinner	Lispro	5 units	Baked potato	6 oz	30
			Chicken breast	4 oz	0
			Dinner rolls	2	30
			Banana–medium	1	30
					Total 90
9:30 P.M.	Glargine	20 units			

Notes about day:

Meet DT

DT is a 34-year-old man who has had type 1 diabetes for fourteen years. He recently started on multiple daily injections of lispro (rapid-acting insulin) at meals and glargine (long-acting insulin) once a day at bedtime. At present, he is using Carb Counting and takes the same amount of lispro with each meal.

STEP 1. FIND THE PATTERNS

DT checks which blood glucose levels are in and out of his target range. He marks them with two different colored highlighters (remember the supply list mentioned before?). His log shows him

			Blood glucose results				
Fasting/ before b'fast/ time	**After b'fast/ time**	**Before lunch/ time**	**After lunch/ time**	**Before dinner/ time**	**After dinner/ time**	**Before bed/ time**	**Other/ time**
Fasting 140 Pre-breakfast 8:15 A.M.	90/ 9:45 A.M.						Aerobics 1 hr after breakfast
		75/ 1:55 P.M.	120/ 4:00 P.M.				
				100/ 5:15 P.M.	180/ 7:40 P.M.		

that he has a fasting blood glucose of 140 mg/dl. When he goes for an hour of aerobics (four to five times a week before breakfast), his fasting blood glucose is 70 mg/dl, showing the direct effect of exercise on his blood glucose level. He took 5 units of lispro before breakfast. His carbohydrate amount at breakfast was 38 g. Two hours after breakfast it was 90 mg/dl.

He was going to have lunch later than usual at 2 P.M. and was concerned that he would get hypoglycemic waiting that long. So, he ate a chocolate candy bar with 28 g of carbohydrate. He checked his blood glucose before lunch and it was 75 mg/dl. He took 5 units of lispro and ate 60 g of carb. His blood glucose two hours after the meal was 120 mg/dl. Before dinner it was 100 mg/dl, and he had 90 g of carb at dinner. His blood glucose level was 180 mg/dl two hours after dinner. At bedtime he took his once-a-day dose of 20 units of glargine.

STEP 2. OBSERVE THE PATTERNS

Was there a pattern to his blood glucose levels? He needed to keep records for three to seven days to see a pattern. When he did, he reviewed his blood glucose logs and saw the effect of exercise on lowering blood glucose levels, and the effect of delayed meals on possible hypoglycemia. He noticed that lunches of 60 g of carb worked well with 5 units of lispro.

STEP 3. PLAN AND TAKE ACTION

To find his insulin-to-carb (I:Carb) ratio, he divided the 60 g of carbohydrate by 5 units of lispro. The answer, 12, means that he can take 1 unit of lispro for every 12 g of carbohydrate that he eats. This is called an I:Carb ratio. He can try this ratio for each meal, keep BG logs before and after each meal, and collect some more data to see if it works for every meal. He may need to adjust the I:Carb ratio for breakfast on the days that he does one hour of aerobics, because he'll need less insulin. His health care provider suggested that a new ratio of 1 unit of lispro for every 15 g of carbohydrate may work better.

DT has heard and read more and more about an insulin pump. He has decided to attend a local insulin pump support group to learn more about the various pumps and talk to people who are on them. He realized that the insulin pump is probably just what he needs to match his need for flexibility in his life.

Meet Larry   Larry is a 35-year-old construction worker with type 1 diabetes, who works Monday through Friday. He takes five injections of insulin a day, two of which are Lantus (one in the morning and one before bed). Then he takes aspart (rapid-acting insulin) before each meal based on his blood glucose result and the amount of carbohydrate he will eat at a meal. He has worked with Advanced Carb Counting for some time. His target blood glucose levels before meals are 110 mg/dl and two hours after a meal are 180 mg/dl. He eats about 70–90 g of carbohydrate per meal. He feels he needs even more flexibility in managing his diabetes because the amount of activity he gets varies from day to day, and his weekdays are quite different from his weekends. In addition, he just attended a local insulin pump support group and talked to some people who are on insulin pumps. They all encouraged him to progress his diabetes management to a pump. They all noted that the pump provided them a new level of flexibility and improved control. Larry has talked to his doctor about his desire for a pump. The doctor said that his health plan will require him to provide some blood glucose records among some other items.

STEP 1. FIND THE PATTERNS

He needs to check which blood glucose levels are out of target range. The blood glucose level before lunch is on the low end at 78 mg/dl. His blood glucose two hours after lunch is also lower than his target of 180 mg/dl. His blood glucose before his evening meal is 150 mg/dl, 200 mg/dl before his bedtime snack, and 250 mg/dl before bedtime.

STEP 2. OBSERVE THE PATTERNS

He tries to find the reasons for the highs and lows. The log shows that the lunch meal was at 1:30 P.M., and breakfast was at 8 A.M., which was a long time in between. Breakfast was only 69 g of carb, but close to the target of 70–90 g. Also there was a lot of physical activity at work. So, there are a few variables to look at. He ate enough carbohydrate, but the lunch meal was delayed and the intensity of physical activity was high. All of these contributed

Larry's Carbohydrate Counting and Blood Glucose Results Record

Day/Date: *Wednesday*

Time/ meal	Diabetes medicines		Food		Carb count (servings/ grams)
	Type	Amount	Type	Amount	
7:00 A.M.	Lantus	16 u			
8:00 A.M.	Humalog	5 u	Egg McMuffins	2	54
			Orange juice	1 cup	30
					Total 84
1:30 P.M.	Humalog	5 u	Cheeseburger	1	28
			Fries	Medium	43
			Diet soda	12 oz	0
					Total 71
4:00 P.M.	Humalog	4 u	Chocolate chip cookie	Large	50 (from label)
6:30 P.M.	Humalog	8 u	Steak	8 oz	0
			Baked potato	6 oz	30
			Corn	1 cup	30
			Dinner roll	2	30
					Total 90
9:30 P.M.			Ice cream	1 cup	30

Notes about day:

			Blood glucose results				
Fasting/ before b'fast/ time	After b'fast/ time	Before lunch/ time	After lunch/ time	Before dinner/ time	After dinner/ time	Before bed/ time	Other/ time
120 (7:50 A.M.)							Went to work Physical activity
		78 (1:25 P.M.)					
			80 (3:30 P.M.)				
							Worked construction
				150 (6:20 P.M.)			Watched TV
					200 (8:30 P.M.)	250 (11:00 P.M.)	Watched TV

Larry's Pump Record

Larry was able to move from his 5 shot a day plan with Lantus and mealtime aspart insulin to an insulin pump. These are four days of records after Larry was on his pump for about two months. He finally got his basal rates for the weekdays and weekends set, and he is feeling that his control is improving. He is thrilled with his new flexibility and better control. He does realize, however, how much more effort is required to use an insulin pump correctly.

Day/Date (fill in times)	12A	3A	6A	B'4 Meal/B	2 hr aft. Meal	Other	B'4 Meal/L	2 hr aft. Meal	Other	B'4 Meal/D	2 hr aft. Meal	Other HS
Blood glucose	160	115	122	128	160		90	178		130	175	158
Carb grams				70			60			80		
Insulin (rapid-acting) to cover carb				4.6			4			53		
Insulin (rapid-acting) to cover high BG				.2						.3		.5

Day/Date (fill in times)	12A	3A	6A	B'4 Meal/B	2 hr aft. Meal	Other	B'4 Meal/L	2 hr aft. Meal	Other	B'4 Meal/D	2 hr aft. Meal	Other HS
Blood glucose	150	125	120	124	111		80	168		112	170	130
Carb grams				80			75			87		—
Insulin (rapid-acting) to cover carb				5.3			5			5.8		—
Insulin (rapid-acting) to cover high BG				—			—1			—.1		—

Day/Date (fill in times)	12A	3A	6A	B'4 Meal/B	2 hr aft. Meal	Other	B'4 Meal/L	2 hr aft. Meal	Other	B'4 Meal/D	2 hr aft. Meal	Other HS
Blood glucose	140	118	114	120	130		111	160		120	178	200
Carb grams				90			75			100		
Insulin (rapid-acting) to cover carb				6			5			6.6		2
Insulin (rapid-acting) to cover high BG				–			–.2			–		2

Day/Date (fill in times)	12A	3A	6A	B'4 Meal/B	2 hr aft. Meal	Other	B'4 Meal/L	2 hr aft. Meal	Other	B'4 Meal/D	2 hr aft. Meal	Other HS
Blood glucose	175	150	140	138	185		103			122	170	115
Carb grams				92			100			90		35
Insulin (rapid-acting) to cover carb				6.1			6.6			6		2.1
Insulin (rapid-acting) to cover high BG				.1			–.1					.4

to the blood glucose of 78 mg/dl before lunch, even though he had started the day with a blood glucose of 120 mg/dl, close to target range. His blood glucose two hours after lunch was 80 mg/dl, as he continued physical work. He had eaten his target carbohydrate at his lunch meal, but his two-hour blood glucose of 80 mg/dl after the lunch meal was much lower than his target blood glucose of 180 mg/dl after a meal. This could have been due to the intensity of the physical activity at work. He needs to eat more carb at breakfast and lunch. The pattern during the day was BG levels on the low side compared to his targets for the day. However, his evening BG levels were higher than his target, perhaps from the carbohydrate in the cookie he ate mid-afternoon and from dinner and the ice cream before bedtime.

STEP 3. PLAN AND TAKE ACTION

Larry and his doctor talked more about his desire to move to an insulin pump. Larry had done his homework by having a representative from each of the pump companies come talk to him about their pump. He asked his doctor also for his recommendation. Larry decided on a particular pump due to its features and the feeling that he got from the company representatives he had met with and spoke with. His doctor submitted the necessary forms to his health plan. Larry was approved for a pump. The company told him to expect his pump in a few weeks and he would be contacted by a pump trainer who would meet with him soon. He would need some more training on Advanced Carb Counting and all the aspects of his pump.

Don't Check Lots, Check Smart

Hopefully through reviewing these sample records you are beginning to understand the value of record keeping and pattern management. The frequency with which you check your blood glucose and keep records will vary based on your needs and desires, whether you have or need to make an adjustment in your regimen, and whether you regularly adjust your insulin doses based on your results. Some people with type 2 diabetes on one type of medication check their blood glucose two to three times a day a few times a week. Some people with type 1 diabetes on an insulin pump check their blood glucose upwards of six times a day every day. No matter how often you check, keep in mind that you want to check smart versus a lot. Checking smart means checking strategically. Always have in mind why and what you are checking and what information this check will provide. Yes, blood glucose monitoring and record keeping is an investment of time and energy, but it can pay big dividends in day-to-day and long-term health.

12

Ready, Willing, and Able to Progress?

It's Time to Assess Yourself

Now it's time to determine whether you need or want to progress from Basic Carb Counting to Advanced Carb Counting. Whether you need to progress to Advanced Carb Counting, as you have likely surmised by now, is related to the diabetes medicines you take, how intensively you need or want to manage your blood glucose levels, and your desire for flexibility in your lifestyle.

If you have type 2 diabetes and manage your blood glucose levels with a steady dose of one or more oral diabetes medicines then you can continue to use Basic Carb Counting. Consistently check your blood glucose levels, do pattern management, and, if your blood glucose levels start to trend upward, consult with your health care provider. Today it is well known that type 2 diabetes progresses over time. What that means is that as the years go by your body loses its ability to secrete insulin from your pancreas. Nearly 50–60% of people with type 2 diabetes eventually need to take insulin by injection or pump to control their blood glucose levels.

Maybe you have had type 2 diabetes for more than fifteen years and your health care provider is suggesting that you have reached that point where you need several insulin injections a day. Or maybe you have type 1 diabetes and have just switched to use a newer insulin regimen with four or five shots a day (a long-acting insulin with a rapid-acting mealtime insulin) or you want to move towards an insulin pump. If you are in one of these situations you could gain flexibility and better control of your blood glucose levels with Advanced Carb Counting. But first, you will want to do a self-assessment to determine if you are ready, willing, and able to progress to Advanced Carb Counting. See if any of the following apply to you and your situation.

1. You cannot achieve your target blood glucose goals with Basic Carb Counting.

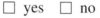 yes □ no

2. You have determined that your lifestyle and eating habits just don't conform to set times and amounts of foods each day. You have learned that you want and need more flexibility in your diabetes plan.

□ yes □ no

3. You have gained an understanding of the benefits of a four-to-five-shot-a-day insulin regimen or an insulin pump and you are willing to do the extra work to gain the flexibility and better control.

□ yes □ no

4. You can and are willing to, several times a day, do the math in order to make adjustments in the amount of insulin you take based on your personalized Advanced Carb Counting factors.

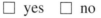 yes □ no

5. You are willing and able to check your blood glucose levels at least four times each day in order to figure the amount of mealtime insulin to take based on the amount of carbohydrate you will eat and your current blood glucose level.

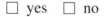 yes □ no

6. You are willing to take the time to analyze your blood glucose results and review patterns and other factors to continue to fine-tune your diabetes plan over time.

☐ yes   ☐ no

7. You have a diabetes care provider who is willing to help you transition to an intensive diabetes management plan and able to help you develop the skills to practice Advanced Carb Counting.

☐ yes   ☐ no

If you can answer "yes" to all of these statements, then you are likely ready to progress to Advanced Carb Counting.

Meet Bob

Bob has had type 2 diabetes for about seventeen years. He is 67 now and has been retired for two years from his career as an engineer. For the first ten or so years he had diabetes, he really didn't pay much attention to it other than to take his diabetes pills. He monitored his blood glucose just when he thought it might be too high, but not regularly. He didn't pay too much attention to what he was eating and when.

Unfortunately, Bob recently began seeing spots in one of his eyes. It was diagnosed as diabetic retinopathy. He had some laser surgery to delay its further progression. This made Bob realize that he had better start paying more attention to his diabetes if he wanted to keep seeing and keep other parts of his body healthy. He started monitoring his blood glucose levels more often and realized that they are often over 200 mg/dl, and many of them are even higher. His doctor recently suggested that he should start to take insulin to get his blood glucose levels back in control. Bob knew this day was coming. He tried to put it off as long as he could. Bob's doctor started him on some bedtime Lantus insulin—the long-acting insulin. His doctor also referred him to a dietitian to learn Advanced Carb Counting. His doctor said that Bob would need to add the mealtime rapid-acting insulin in amounts based on his mealtime blood glucose level and the amount of carb he was going to eat. This was why he really needed to learn Advanced Carb Counting.

At Bob's first visit with the dietitian they talked about what Bob was willing to do to take care of his diabetes. The dietitian let Bob know that making decisions about how much insulin to take before meals takes effort and some mathematics. Since Bob now had a bit of time on his hands and was an engineer for many years, he knew he could handle the math and wanted this more precise way of managing his blood glucose levels. He decided to give it a try. The dietitian told Bob that they would start with the basics about carbohydrates and determine how much carbohydrate he wanted and needed at each of his meals. She explained how the amount of rapid-acting insulin he took at meals would be determined by two things—what Bob's blood glucose was before his meal and what he planned to eat. The dietitian told Bob that he should return for several visits to make sure he understood how to do this and to fine-tune his control. Bob left the dietitian's office with a better understanding of what foods contain carbohydrate. He also had a basic plan for how many carb choices or grams of carbohydrate he needed at breakfast, lunch, and dinner. In addition, Bob knew that he would start using an insulin-to-carbohydrate (I:Carb) ratio of 1:15, or 1 unit of rapid-acting insulin to cover each 15 grams (g) of carbohydrate. The key now was to follow this meal plan carefully, which included weighing and measuring his foods for a while and monitoring his blood glucose both before and after his meals. Checking his blood glucose was the only way to fine-tune his I:Carb ratio so it worked for him. Before leaving, Bob made the next appointment with the dietitian for 2 weeks later. She asked him to remember to bring in his food and blood glucose records for the visit. She also encouraged him to bring in food labels from foods he usually ate and a list of the foods he typically eats when he dines out. They will figure out how he can fit these foods into his carbohydrate counting plan, too.

13

Advanced Carb Counting
ALL THE INS AND OUTS

Guess your self-assessment from chapter 12 led you to realize that you want and need to progress to Advanced Carb Counting. Perhaps you are just transitioning to multiple insulin injections from oral medicines and one nighttime insulin injection, or from multiple injections to an insulin pump. Or maybe you are tired of the giant blood glucose roller coaster you've been on and are looking for a sensible and flexible approach to managing your blood glucose levels. Whatever reason you have, congratulations on taking this step towards better control of your blood glucose and diabetes. You'll find that many diabetes health providers refer to a diabetes management plan that includes multiple injections or an insulin pump with Advanced Carb Counting as intensive diabetes management.

This chapter gives you an orientation to the terms of Advanced Carb Counting. With these terms you will learn how to figure a couple of factors that you will use to calculate your rapid-acting insulin doses. You'll learn how to personalize these factors for you and how to adjust them over time. There is a lot to learn, and it's important that you take it one step at a time. You'll likely have many questions as you read through this chapter. So, the next chapter, chapter 14, provides answers to the most commonly asked questions about Advanced Carb Counting.

As you move forward, please recognize that Advanced Carb Counting and the adjustment of insulin is not a do-it-yourself activity. The body is very complex, and each person with diabetes is unique. We encourage you to find and work closely with diabetes care providers who are knowledgeable about intensive diabetes management. Find providers who are willing to give you the time you need to develop and apply the ratios, as well as work with you to fine-tune your control and make adjustments as your diabetes and your lifestyle change.

Why the Giant Roller Coaster Ride?

One reason you may experience large swings in your blood glucose is that you may be caught in the vicious cycle of treating high blood glucose levels that have already occurred—think of this as "retrospective management." What you've been doing is trying to lower a high blood glucose that has occurred due to a situation during the last few hours—for instance, excess carbohydrate or insufficient insulin—with insulin that works in the future (over the next few hours). This scenario keeps you on a roller coaster ride. And you can't get off unless you change your ways and learn to do "prospective management," as you'll learn in this chapter. Getting off the giant roller coaster and onto a more reasonable ride means you will learn to take insulin in sync with the amount of carbohydrate you eat as well as other factors.

Let's look at this critical concept up close. Many people who take rapid-acting insulin several times a day at meals are provided by their health care provider with a formula with which to calculate their mealtime insulin doses. For example, you might have been told to take 5 units of insulin if your blood glucose is between 150 and 200 mg/dl, 7 units of insulin if your blood glucose is between 200 and 250 mg/dl, and so on. There are three basic flaws with this method:

1. It is treating a high blood glucose (something that has occurred over the previous few hours) with rapid-acting

insulin that has its action in the future—over the next three to five hours. This simply isn't going to work.

2. This formula doesn't factor in how much carbohydrate you will eat. It is simply focused on the result of your blood glucose from the past few hours. This just doesn't make sense because the amount of carbohydrate you eat is the biggest predictor of how much your blood glucose will rise during the next few hours.

3. Many people—but certainly not everyone—require about 1 unit of insulin to decrease blood glucose by 50 mg/dl. Therefore, a fifty-point spread could be the difference of needing 1 or 2 units of insulin—too big of a spread for intensive diabetes management.

For the above reasons, we encourage you to do prospective management of your blood glucose—look forward. And that's what you'll learn in this chapter. You'll learn to factor in both your mealtime blood glucose level and the amount of carbohydrate you will eat at the meal. Obviously, it's also good to consider other things that will occur over the next few hours that affect your blood glucose, such as your level of activity. For instance, are you going to take a longer than usual walk or be less active than usual? The more prospective—future oriented—you can be in your estimation of your insulin needs, the better your control will be.

A New Vocabulary

To do Advanced Carb Counting, you'll need to master a new lexicon. Let's define these.

Basal insulin. The pancreas of a person who does not have diabetes puts out about 1 unit of insulin per hour, whether or not you eat any food. This is simply the amount of insulin the body needs hour to hour to keep functioning properly and to supply glucose to the cells. If you take insulin, basal insulin is what you need to keep your blood glucose level in control, regardless of whether you eat any food. Another term you might hear used for basal insulin is *background insulin.*

The preferred insulin used for basal insulin has changed over the last few years. Before 2001 NPH, lente, and ultralente were the only long-acting insulins available to serve as basal insulin. It didn't do a great job, but it was all that was available. As of 2001 in the U.S., glargine, brand name Lantus, was approved. Another longer-acting insulin, Detemer, is expected shortly. If you currently use an intermediate-acting insulin (NPH or lente) or the long-acting insulin (ultralente), you might want to talk to your diabetes care provider about making a change to a true long-acting insulin. Look at Table 13-1 to see the action times of insulins and Figure 13-1 to see the action curves of the different types of insulin. People on an insulin pump set basal rates for insulin, however all of the insulin used in an insulin pump is most often one type of rapid-acting insulin that is constantly administered in small amounts over a long period of time.

Establishing the amount of basal insulin that you need from a long-acting insulin is not simple. That's in part because of the possible ups and downs of blood glucose levels during the day and night. For example, some people's blood glucose levels go up

TABLE 13-1 The Action of Insulins

Insulin	Onset	Peak	Duration
Rapid acting			
lispro (Humalog)	<15 minutes	0.5–1.5 hours	2–4 hours
aspart (Novolog)	<15 minutes	0.5–1.0 hour	1–3 hours
Short acting			
regular	0.5–1 hour	2–3 hours	3–6 hours
Intermediate			
NPH	2–4 hours	4–10 hours	10–16 hours
lente	3–4 hours	4–12 hours	12–18 hours
Long acting			
ultralente	6–10 hours	10–16 hours	18–20 hours
glargine (Lantus)	2–4 hours	peakless	24 hours

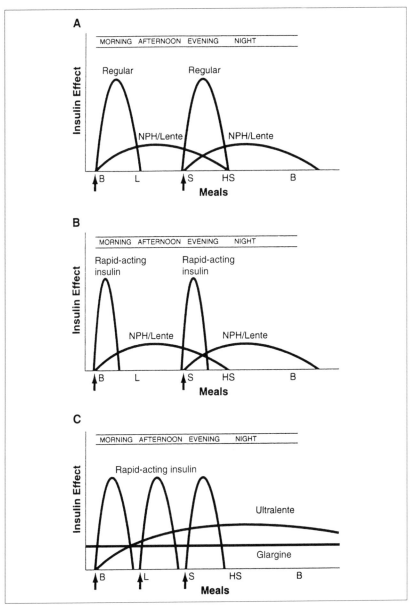

Figure 13-1   **(A)** Short-acting and intermediate-acting insulin.
(B) Rapid-acting and intermediate-acting insulin. (B = breakfast,
L = lunch, S = supper, HS = evening snack, B = bedtime)
(C) Rapid-acting with meals and long-acting insulin in the
evening. (B = breakfast, L = lunch, S = supper, HS = evening
snack, B = bedtime)

before they wake due to a rise in hormones at that time of day. This is called the *dawn phenomenon* and may require more insulin to achieve blood glucose targets. Some people's blood glucose levels tend to track downward in the early hours of the night, thus they need less insulin during that time frame.

All this is to say that there are many variables to consider as you fine-tune your background insulin. It is also why some people choose an insulin pump. Most insulin pumps allow you to have different basal rates during the 24 hours of the day. They also allow you to have different basal rates for different days of the week—for weekday and weekend variation, for days you run and days you don't, etc. This is one huge plus of an insulin pump.

Generally, about 50% of your total insulin intake in 24 hours will be your basal insulin, but you might find you need as little as 45% (or less) or as much as 60% (or more).

Bolus insulin. When people who don't have diabetes eat, their bodies automatically put the amount of insulin they need into the bloodstream to keep blood glucose under about 140 mg/dl. Bolus insulin is the amount of rapid- or short-acting insulin that you need to "cover" the amount of food—especially carbohydrate—that you eat. This is the insulin you need to bring your blood glucose back to premeal target levels within about three to four hours after the start of a meal. Bolus insulin can account for as little as 40% (or less) of the total daily insulin dose or as much as 55% (or more). You use your I:Carb ratio to calculate your bolus insulin doses.

Insulin-to-carb (I:Carb) ratio. An I:Carb ratio tells you the amount of rapid-acting bolus insulin you need to "cover" the amount of carbohydrate you eat to bring your blood glucose level back to premeal target levels within about three to four hours after you start to eat. In the next few pages you'll learn a couple of methods to calculate an I:Carb ratio that you can start with. Some diabetes health care providers just start people off with an I:Carb of

1:15. This would mean that you take 1 unit of rapid-acting insulin for every 15 grams (g) of carbohydrate you eat. For example, your meal has 72 g of carb. To find out how much insulin you need to take to cover it, you divide the grams of carb in the meal by the number of carbs covered by 1 unit of insulin.

72 g ÷ 15 = 4.8, or round up (if you aren't on a pump) to 5

This means you need to take 5 units of rapid-acting insulin to cover the carbohydrate in this meal. When you use I:Carb ratios to figure your bolus insulin doses, you can be more flexible about what and how much you eat—and when you eat, too.

People who are sensitive to insulin—meaning that small amounts of insulin lower their blood glucose rapidly—might need a higher I:Carb ratio, such as 1:20. On the other hand, people who are insensitive to insulin—meaning it takes a lot of insulin to lower their blood glucose—might need a lower insulin-to-carb ratio, such as 1:10.

To make things even more interesting, you might find that you need to use different I:Carb ratios at different times of the day. For example, some people who eat the same amount of carb at breakfast, lunch, and dinner need more insulin in the morning than they do at lunch or dinner. That might be because they are more insulin resistant in the morning due to the influence of the hormones that wake you up.

Postprandial blood glucose (PPG). Postprandial blood glucose is your blood glucose level after you eat. It is formally defined by the American Diabetes Association (ADA) as two hours after the start of a meal. Checking your PPG when you do Advanced Carb Counting is critical. It's the only way to see how well your bolus doses and your I:Carb ratios work. The ADA target for PPG 180 mg/dl or less.

Multiple daily injections (MDIs). People who take insulin and want to control their blood glucose levels closely take multiple daily insulin injections. Today that means four to five shots—one or two shots of a longer-acting insulin (Lantus) and three shots at or around meals. (Another long-acting insulin, Detemer, from Novo Nordisk Pharmaceuticals, will be added soon. However, the dosing will be different.)

Insulin pump. The type of insulin pumps available today are called "open-loop pumps." An insulin pump is a small device about the size of a pager. Very thin plastic tubing runs from the syringe in the pump to a very fine tube that is inserted under the skin in the abdomen or another place that is comfortable for you. Pumps can hold enough insulin to last two to three days. With assistance from your pump trainer and diabetes care providers, you "program" the pump to provide both basal and bolus insulin. Basal insulin is provided in continuous tiny amounts over 24 hours. You can adjust the basal amount in various ways with most pumps to get more or less basal insulin during a 24-hour period. You decide how much bolus insulin to take by checking your premeal blood glucose. Then you determine how much carb you will eat. All in all, the insulin pump delivers insulin in a way that more closely mimics a normal pancreas.

In the near future it is likely that "closed loop" pumps will automatically check your blood glucose with a sensor that is part of the system. Using your blood glucose results, the pump would automatically give you the amount of insulin you need.

How to Determine Your I:Carb Ratio

Now that you have the Advanced Carb Counting terms under your belt, let's move on to ways you can determine your insulin-to-carb ratios. As a word of caution, always be conservative. You don't want to take too much insulin because you don't want to increase your frequency of hypoglycemia. Work out your I:Carb ratios with the advice of your diabetes care provider.

METHOD #1: USE YOUR FOOD DIARY AND BLOOD GLUCOSE RECORDS

You can use the food and blood glucose record that we've used through the book (a blank is in Appendix 3) or a form that you have developed. You need a record of at least several days, but a whole week is even better. Be sure to track the grams of carb you eat, the amount of rapid- or short-acting insulin you take before the meal, and your blood glucose results. Note whenever your blood glucose is too high or too low. It is helpful to do more blood glucose checks during this phase—both before you eat and two hours after you start to eat to get your PPG. All this information will help you establish a more precise I:Carb ratio. While you're compiling your daily records, it is a good idea to try and keep your carb grams and the amount of activity you do as consistent as possible.

Next, study your records. Then, using the methods reviewed in chapter 11, calculate your I:Carb ratio. For each meal or snack you ate, divide the total grams of carb by the number of units of rapid- or short-acting insulin you took to achieve your target blood glucose level. You might find that you need different insulin-to-carb ratios for different times of the day. You might also find that you need different amounts of insulin for certain foods or meals, such as pizza, a high-protein and high-fat meal, or for prolonged meals, such as a buffet dinner party.

Example: Look first at breakfasts. You see that generally you eat about 60 g of carb, and you take about 4 units of rapid-acting insulin. This amount of insulin seems to get you back to your pre-meal target blood glucose within three and a half hours. That's good. To find a breakfast I:Carb ratio, you divide 60 g carb by 4 units insulin. The answer is 15, or 1 unit of insulin for every 15 g of carbohydrate—an insulin-to-carb ratio of 1:15.

Method #1 will work if your blood glucose level is generally within your targets both before and after eating. If you are not near your targets, this method will not be as helpful because the amount of insulin you are taking is not achieving good blood glucose control. If this is the case, method #2 might work better as a starting point.

METHOD #2: THE GUIDELINE OF 500

In this chapter we'll introduce you to two "guidelines." You'll learn how to personalize each for you. These guidelines are based on the clinical experience and research of a number of diabetes experts who have worked with many people with diabetes who use intensive diabetes management. Today these guidelines are well accepted in the diabetes community. Two people who should be mentioned by name for their contributions to this area are John Walsh, PA, CDE, the author of the book *Pumping Insulin*, (noted on page 200 in the pump resources) and Paul Davidson, MD, an endocrinologist in Atlanta, Georgia.

The first—the guideline of 500—can be used to calculate your starting insulin-to-carb ratios. The 500 guideline is useful to determine your initial I:Carb ratio if you take rapid-acting insulin. Some clinicians use 450 to calculate the I:Carb ratio if you take short-acting insulin.

Here's how to use it: First find your Total Daily Dose (TDD) of insulin. You find your TDD by adding all the insulin you take in 24 hours—both rapid and longer acting. Then simply divide the number 500 by your TDD of insulin.

Example: Let's say your TDD is 42 units.

$$500 \div 42 = 12$$

This means your I:Carb ratio is 1:12, or 1 unit of rapid-acting insulin for every 12 g carbohydrate you eat in a meal or snack.

Now, you have an insulin-to-carb ratio of 1:12. Let's say you eat a breakfast that has 60 g carb in it. How much insulin are you going to take to cover the carb in the meal? Divide the total carb in the meal by the number of carb grams 1 unit of insulin will cover.

60 g ÷ 12 = 5 units of insulin

You will take 5 units of insulin to cover the 60 g carb meal.

Compare the Methods to Determine Insulin-to-Carb Ratios

Check it out. Did you get the same I:Carb ratio using method #1 that you got with method #2? Are they close or far apart? The only way to check whether the I:Carb ratio works for you is to use it and check your blood glucose levels frequently. You will soon learn whether it works for you or you will have the information to figure a new insulin-to-carb ratio.

Calculating a Sensitivity Factor

So, you know how to figure how much mealtime insulin to take to cover carbs. But what should you do if your blood glucose is higher than your premeal target when you eat your meal? You need to use a second factor—your sensitivity factor (SF). Note that another term is used for this factor—correction factor. They mean the same thing. The SF tells you how much additional rapid-acting insulin you need to get your blood glucose back to your premeal target level or how many points 1 unit of rapid-acting insulin will lower your blood glucose level. Your SF, as you can imagine, will depend on how sensitive you are to insulin.

This is where the second guideline of this chapter comes in. The guideline of 1800 is a method to calculate how much 1 unit of rapid-acting insulin lowers your blood glucose. Here's how it works. As with the guideline of 500, you need to figure your TDD of insulin. Then divide 1800 by your TDD to determine your correction factor.

Example: Let's say your TDD is 35.

$1800 \div 35 = 51$ (round it to 50)

This means that 1 unit of rapid-acting insulin lowers blood glucose by 50 mg/dl, and your sensitivity factor is 1 to 50. Some clinicians find that using the number 1500 is more accurate for people who take short-acting insulin.

Now that you have an SF, let's try to figure out a hypothetical correction dose. You check your blood glucose before dinner, and it is 225 mg/dl. Your target premeal blood glucose level is 110 mg/dl. To find out how much you need to lower your blood glucose to get to your target, you subtract the target level from the actual blood glucose.

225 (actual blood glucose) – 110 (target premeal blood glucose) = 125 (the difference between where you are and where you want to be)

We figured out above that your (theoretical) SF is 1–50. If you take 1 unit of insulin to lower your blood glucose by 50 mg/dl, how many units of insulin do you need to lower it by 125 mg/dl?

$125 \div 50 = 2.5$ units of insulin

There you go. Using your SF you see that you need to take 2 1/2 units of insulin to get your blood glucose to target levels. If you take insulin via injections or pens that count in whole numbers, round down to 2. If you use a pump you can take the exact dose.

If your premeal target is a range of 90–130 mg/dl, then you can select a number within that range to use as your premeal target. You have to have one number to use in this formula (as above). You may want to use the midpoint of 110 or 120 mg/dl.

Figuring Your Insulin Dose

Using the two guidelines in the previous examples, we have found that you need 5 units of insulin to cover the 60 g of carbohydrate in your breakfast. You also need 2 units of insulin to bring your blood glucose back to your premeal target. So, to figure how much rapid-acting insulin to take, you add the two results:

5 units for the meal + 2 units to correct = 7 units of insulin

Here's another opportunity for you to practice. Try to figure out a dose using the following information:

- Premeal blood glucose is 175 mg/dl

- Target premeal blood glucose is 120 mg/dl

- Sensitivity factor is 1 unit to lower blood glucose 70 mg/dl

- Amount of carb in meal is 69 g

- Insulin-to-carb ratio is 1:16

Let's get started. First, we'll figure out how much we need to lower the blood glucose level.

175 (actual blood glucose) – 120 (target premeal blood glucose) = 55 mg/dl

Using the SF, we need to figure out how much insulin is needed to get levels into target range.

55 ÷ 70 (the SF) = 0.8 unit of insulin (round up to 1 if not on an insulin pump)

So it will take 1 unit of insulin to correct the premeal glucose level. Now we need to figure out how much insulin to use to cover the carbohydrate in the meal. The I:Carb ratio is 1:16.

69 g carb ÷ 16 = 4.3, or round down to 4 units of insulin

Now you add the correction insulin to the meal insulin.

1 unit + 4 units = 5 units

There you go. You take 5 units of premeal bolus insulin to cover the meal.

It's important to look at the patterns of your blood glucose. If day after day you have to use one or several units of insulin to correct your blood glucose level before a meal, then you either need more basal insulin in the time leading up to that meal or you need to increase the bolus insulin for the previous meal. Use the information you gain from having to use sensitivity factors to make finer adjustments to your insulin doses and be within your target ranges all day long.

What about a Premeal Low Blood Glucose?

If your blood glucose happens to be too low (less than 70 mg/dl before a meal), you need to factor this into your mealtime insulin. Obviously, hypoglycemia isn't always going to conveniently happen just before meal time, but for the sake of this explanation. . .

You have two options:

1. **Take less insulin.** Using the same numbers from the example above, you would subtract 1 unit of insulin from the mealtime dose and only take 4 units of insulin for the 69 g of carb. This is the preferred option, especially if you are watching your weight and very conscious of your calorie intake.
2. **Eat more carbohydrate at the meal.** In the example above, you could add another 15 g of carb to the 69 g in the meal but not take any more insulin. The extra 15 g of carb would work to raise blood glucose.

What you definitely don't want to do is not take the mealtime insulin or delay the mealtime insulin a lot. Once the carb you eat starts to enter your body, your blood glucose will rise and you will need insulin to cover the rise. With experimentation you will learn whether one way works better than another for you. In these situations, be alert for signs of hypoglycemia and treat it as soon as it is coming on.

If you have frequent high or low premeal blood glucose levels, then you need to check your basal dose, too. It might be too high, causing the premeal lows. Work with your diabetes care providers to help you make the needed adjustments to get your numbers closer to target.

When to Take Mealtime Insulin—Before, During, or After?

The answer? All of the above! However, you have likely heard health care providers tell you to take your rapid-acting insulin *before* you eat. Why is this? It's likely because prior to the days of rapid-acting insulin, the insulin that was used to cover the rise of blood glucose from meals was regular insulin. For regular insulin to have a snowball's chance in you-know-where of covering the rise of blood glucose from meals, it was important to take it thirty minutes prior to the meal.

Now that rapid-acting insulin is available, the advice can be quite different. Plus, the reality is that there are times in your life when you know exactly how much carb you will eat and others when you don't have a clue. Take for instance breakfast. You know how much cereal and milk you will pour in the bowl and you know that you will eat it all. Conversely, there are times when you may be in a new restaurant or feeling a bit under the weather. At these times, you won't know how much carb you will eat until your meal is complete.

A note to parents with young children and/or finicky eaters: It will likely relieve a lot of stress at mealtimes for you to give your child their mealtime rapid-acting insulin dose after your child has finished eating. This way you can count up the amount of carb your child has eaten and give the right amount of insulin to cover. You will no longer have to force-feed your child because you have already given a fixed amount of insulin.

From a practical standpoint, the best approach to use when trying to decide when to take rapid-acting mealtime insulin is to take your insulin **when you *know* how much carbohydrate you will eat or have eaten.** So, there are times when you might take it just before you sit down to eat and others halfway during the meal and yet others when you have finished a meal. Using this strategy can help you better estimate the amount of insulin you need and to avoid under- or overestimates.

There are a few more tricks to take advantage of if you are on an insulin pump or if you don't mind an extra injection. (The beauty of a pump is that it's just the press of a button and not another injection.) If your blood glucose is higher than your pre-meal target, you can take the amount of insulin you need based on your sensitivity factor to bring you down to your mealtime target. Then if you don't know how much carb you will eat you can wait until the end of the meal to cover your carb based on your I:Carb ratio. There's also another trick to play with split mealtime doses. If you know you will eat at least a certain amount of carb in a meal and you know your blood glucose rises fairly quickly after you start to eat, you can give yourself a certain amount of insulin to start working. Then after the meal you can take an additional bolus dose to cover the amount of carb you ate in excess of what you covered at the beginning of the meal.

Most of the insulin pumps have ways in which you can split your mealtime insulin dose with a square wave bolus, also called extended bolus; or dual wave or combo bolus, also accomplished with a normal bolus plus extended bolus.

Don't Forget to Factor in Insulin on Board

If you take multiple daily insulin injections or are on an insulin pump, you'll want to pay careful attention to the amount of insulin that you still have "on board," or that is unused, from the last bolus dose prior to deciding on your next bolus dose. Unfortunately, this is a concept that is often overlooked and one that, if not addressed, can lead to too much hypoglycemia. This is to prevent so-called "overlapping" or "stacking" insulin doses. Keep in mind that this is not a problem for everyone. It is more of a problem for people in whom rapid-acting insulin takes longer to complete its action, at least more than four hours.

To further explain this concept, consider this example. You take a lunchtime bolus dose of rapid-acting insulin. Then three hours later you choose to have a snack with 35 g of carbohydrate. You check your blood glucose and it's 195 mg/dl. You want to bring that 195 mg/dl down, so you take 2 units of insulin to bring you back down to your premeal target of 120 mg/dl and you take 2 units to cover the carb. Several hours later your blood glucose is 55 mg/dl. Why? It's because you "stacked your insulin." You didn't factor in that at three hours into the action of your lunchtime rapid-acting bolus there was still at least one hour of action left on that insulin—you had "unused insulin" or "insulin on board." That insulin you took for lunch was still in your body and hadn't completely acted.

So, when you take rapid-acting insulin with each meal you need to be certain that when you take your next bolus dose that the previous bolus dose has completed its action (by about four or five hours). Or if you believe that the previous bolus dose still has some action time, then you account for the as yet "unused insulin" or "insulin on board." You also need to use this thinking if your blood glucose is higher than you want it to be within about four hours after a meal and you want to take additional insulin to bring it down. John Walsh, PA, CDE, and author of *Pumping Insulin* feels that about 30% of a dose of Humalog or Novolog will be used each hour after it is given.

There are several ways to manage this. The quick and easy way is to use a higher number, such as 180 mg/dl, as your premeal target versus somewhere between 100 and 130 mg/dl. This way you wouldn't have taken any insulin to cover the high and would just have taken the 2 units to cover the carb in the snack.

In *Pumping Insulin* and on his web site *http://diabetesnet.com/ diabetes_control_tips/unused_insulin_rule.php,* John Walsh provides a table that shows the insulin activity at one, two, three, and four hours after bolus doses of insulin from 1 to 10 units.

You can also use this calculation if your blood glucose is still high a few hours after a meal and you want to get your blood glucose down before you eat your next meal in several hours. For example, if it is two hours after your dinner and your blood glucose is higher than you want it to be, correct your blood glucose with additional rapid-acting insulin down to a target of 180 mg/dl (a two hours after eating target), not to 120 mg/dl (a premeal target).

Interestingly, the latest generation of insulin pumps has a built-in feature that helps people consider their previous bolus dose. What happens is that if you asked the pump to provide you with your next bolus dose prior to the last one being used up, it would ask you if you wanted to subtract the amount of insulin still "on board" from the amount you asked it to provide. This is yet another advantage of an insulin pump. They are adding up!

IS AN INSULIN PEN FOR YOU?

Insulin pens are easy to use. You dial the dose, insert the needle, push the button to inject insulin, and hold. Done! If you are on multiple daily injections, an insulin pen is a good option to consider. Insulin pens make it easier to inject anytime, anywhere in your busy day. People who take three or more shots per day like to use them for their convenience and flexibility, even if you only use them at lunchtime. They are the size of a large fountain pen. For reusable pens, you can buy insulin in cartridges instead of vials.

You may want to try a pen if you:

• Vary how much insulin you take based on what you eat

• Want and need the flexibility and convenience of carrying your insulin with you

• Want a quick, easy, and accurate insulin dose

• Don't mind taking extra shots (you can't mix two types of insulin in one pen)

• Have problems drawing up a dose of insulin due to poor eyesight or shaky hands

Discuss switching to a pen with your health care provider. Learn proper use of the pen and pen needles and proper storage for them.

WHAT DO YOU NEED TO KNOW ABOUT NEEDLES, PEN NEEDLES, AND SYRINGES?

When you buy insulin syringes or pen needles, you make decisions about the needle length, the needle gauge, and the size of the syringe. You'll find that syringes and pen needles come in various lengths and gauges. Common syringe sizes are 30 gauge with a short needle and 29 gauge with a standard needle. Common pen needle sizes are 31 gauge with a short needle and 29 gauge with a standard needle.

Needle gauge. Needles are made in four common gauges: 28, 29, 30, and 31. That's the diameter (width) of the needle. The higher the number the thinner the needle. Different companies make needles in different gauges. The thinnest needle on an insulin syringe is 30 gauge; the thinnest pen needle is 31 gauge.

Syringe size. There are three sizes of insulin syringe: 3/10 cc (holds 30 units), 1/2 cc (holds 50 units), and 1 cc (holds 100 units).

If you take:

• Less than 30 units total at one time, use a 3/10 cc syringe

• Between 30 and 50 units total at one time, use a 1/2 cc syringe

• Between 50 and 100 units total at one time, use a 1 cc syringe

On the 3/10 and 1/2 cc syringes, each line equals 1 unit of insulin. On the 1 cc syringe, each line equals 2 units.

14

Common Questions and Answers about Advanced Carb Counting

HOW DO YOU KNOW HOW MUCH INSULIN YOU NEED?

Unfortunately, there's no simple answer to this question. There are many ifs, ands, and buts. Health care providers have a variety of ways of deciding on starting insulin doses. Several diabetes resources suggest that people with type 1 diabetes who are at or around their desired weight will need about 0.2–0.5 units of insulin per pound of body weight per day. For example, a women who weighs 125 pounds might need about 38 units of insulin for her Total Daily Dose (TDD). Then that total dose would need to be divided into doses based on the types of insulin she was going to use.

It is common for adolescents to need more insulin per pound of body weight due to their increased levels of some hormones. It is typical for people with type 2 diabetes, who may be insulin resistant, to need more insulin. Insulin needs can change as you move through different phases of your life or change your lifestyle. For example, adolescents have surging hormones, which can cause higher than usual insulin needs, and women have different insulin needs in different phases of their menstrual cycle or in different trimesters of pregnancy. A man in retirement who takes up a sport such as bicycling and gets into long-distance rides will have different insulin needs than he did before.

And so go the ifs, ands, or buts. Keep in mind that a starting dose of insulin is just that—a place to start. The next step is to use your records to fine-tune your insulin needs and therefore blood glucose results. One word of wisdom with insulin dosing is to always start conservatively. That's true whether you are just starting on insulin or whether you are moving from insulin by injection to an insulin pump. Better to be safe (and not increase the risk of hypoglycemia) than sorry.

HOW OFTEN SHOULD YOU CHANGE YOUR SENSITIVITY FACTOR AND INSULIN-TO-CARB RATIO?

You should change these any time your TDD changes beyond just a few units up or down (plus or minus 5 units). This change in your TDD might be due to a change in your lifestyle. For example, perhaps you decide to start a walking program and you realize that you need less insulin on the days you are active. Or perhaps you have changed the type of insulin you take. Maybe you changed from two shots of NPH to one bedtime shot of Lantus and you find that you need less Lantus than NPH. Whatever the reason, review your two factors. Put your TDD through the calculations provided in chapter 13. Also, examine your blood glucose records to see if you can track what's happening.

HOW CAN YOU KEEP TRACK OF THESE FACTORS?

Make a notation of your sensitivity factor (SF) and insulin-to-carb (I:Carb) ratio in something that is always with you. It may be a piece of paper in your wallet or in your PDA. This way if you forget, you know where to look. Because you will use these factors a number of times each day, it won't take you long to commit them to memory. When you make a change, make these notations.

HOW CAN YOU DO ALL THE MATH?

It is important to have a calculator with you at all times. Most PDAs come with a calculator or you might find a watch that doubles as a calculator.

WHAT IS THE DIFFERENCE BETWEEN USING RAPID-ACTING INSULIN AND SHORT-ACTING INSULIN?

Rapid-acting insulin works more quickly than short-acting regular insulin. The beauty of rapid-acting insulin is that the peak of its action is more likely to coincide with the rise in blood glucose from the food you've eaten—in about one to two hours. As the carb is raising your blood glucose, the rapid-acting insulin is beginning to lower your blood glucose. Regular insulin doesn't peak until three to four hours after the meal and can miss the mark, so to speak. Do keep in mind that rapid-acting insulin was first introduced in 1995. Short-acting insulin is what many health care providers were accustomed to for many years. If you think an insulin regimen that includes rapid-acting insulin would work better for you, talk to your diabetes care provider. Never make this switch on your own.

DO YOU NEED TO EAT SNACKS ON A MULTIPLE DAILY INJECTION REGIMEN OR INSULIN PUMP?

You can snack less often using a multiple daily injection (MDI) regimen or an insulin pump, or you may be able to omit snacks altogether, particularly if you use rapid-acting insulin. Remember that rapid-acting insulin works with the rise of blood glucose from the meal and is gone from the body within three to four hours. So, if you don't want or like to eat snacks, this type of plan may work well for you. If you want to eat snacks because you enjoy them or find that they help you control your blood glucose better, then you need to determine—with blood glucose checks—whether you need more insulin. See chapter 4.

FOR SNACKS IN BETWEEN MEALS OR A BEDTIME SNACK DO YOU NEED TO TAKE MORE INSULIN?

If you take rapid-acting insulin, you may need to take some to cover the carb from the food in an in between meal snack or a bedtime snack, particularly if those snacks are large. If you have different I:Carb ratios for different meals, try using the ratio for the meal closest to the snack. If you take regular insulin, it usually is working hardest within two to three hours of being injected. So you may not need extra insulin because it will still be working when you eat a snack. Again, checking blood glucose levels is the way to decide what works for you and what doesn't.

HOW DOES A HIGH-FAT OR HIGH-PROTEIN MEAL AFFECT THE RISE IN BLOOD GLUCOSE? HOW DOES PIZZA AFFECT BLOOD GLUCOSE? HOW DOES GRAZING AT A COCKTAIL PARTY FOR SEVERAL HOURS AFFECT BLOOD GLUCOSE?

As discussed in chapter 6, the impact of high-fat, high-protein meals may be different for people with type 1 diabetes than for people with insulin-resistant type 2 diabetes. Here's a starting point. If you take rapid- or short-acting insulin, take the insulin based on your blood glucose level and I:Carb ratio. Then check your blood glucose two to three hours after the meal to see if it is in your target range. A high-fat or high-fat/high-protein meal, such as prime rib, may delay stomach emptying and the rise in blood glucose from two hours after the start of the meal to three to five or even more hours after the start of the meal. If you take rapid-acting insulin, it may peak before your blood glucose peaks, and you end up with hypoglycemia. To prevent this, some people take rapid-acting insulin after a high-fat meal, rather than before, or split the dose and take half before and half after the meal. Clearly, checking your blood glucose levels is the only way you will know the effect of these foods and meals on you.

Pizza is a food that is a puzzlement to some people with diabetes. It can cause blood glucose to rise high in some people and it can cause a delayed rise in blood glucose in some people. For starters, make sure to get a solid carb count to decide on the proper amount of rapid-acting insulin to cover the carbs. Use your I:Carb ratio, and check two hours later to see what it does to your blood glucose levels. If there is a lot of meat and cheese on the pizza and/or if your blood glucose wasn't as high yet as you expected, then check your blood glucose again three to five hours after starting the meal. Keep close records the next time you eat pizza, too. This is important information for you—and you'll use it every time you want to eat pizza.

An insulin pump provides you with even more ways to manage these types of meals. You can calculate the bolus insulin dose for the entire meal, and take one-half or two-thirds the dose at the start of the meal. Then, two to three hours later check your blood glucose and, depending on the level, take the rest of the bolus dose. Most pumps have an option that lets you extend the bolus dose of insulin over several hours. Another option with a pump is to use a temporary basal and increase the basal rate for a few hours to help get your blood glucose down. Both of these methods would work well with meals that raise blood glucose more slowly and meals that extend over a longer than usual period of time, such as at Thanksgiving or large dinner parties.

SHOULD YOU ADJUST THE AMOUNT OF RAPID- OR SHORT-ACTING INSULIN YOU TAKE FOR A HIGH-FIBER MEAL?

Yes, if a food or meal (the combination of several foods) has 5 grams (g) or more of fiber, subtract the grams of fiber from the total grams of carbohydrate in the meal. You want to do this because the fiber content of the total carbohydrate is, for the most part, not digested and not absorbed as glucose. Calculate how much rapid- or short-acting insulin to take based on the amount of carb in the meal, minus the grams of dietary fiber.

Here is an example of a high-fiber breakfast:

Food	Fiber	Carb
1 cup high-fiber cereal	6 g	32 g
1 slice whole-grain bread	3 g	12 g
1 cup low-fat milk	0 g	12 g
1 1/4 cup strawberries	2 g	15 g
Total	**11 g**	**71 g**

Subtract the 11 g of fiber from the 71 g of carbohydrate and figure your insulin dose on 60 g carb. Based on an I:Carb ratio of 1:15, the insulin dose would be:

60 ÷ 15 = 4 units of insulin

SHOULD YOU ADJUST THE AMOUNT OF RAPID- OR SHORT-ACTING INSULIN FOR ALCOHOL?

Review general information about alcohol in chapter 6. The general recommendation from diabetes experts today is to consider the calories from alcoholic beverages in addition to your regular eating plan and don't omit carbohydrate to compensate for the extra calories that are mainly contributed by alcohol. This is a precautionary measure because alcohol can cause blood glucose levels to decrease too much if you take insulin. Use this practice with light beer and any type of wine or distilled spirits. Due to the carb count of regular beer—about 15 g of carb per 12 ounces (oz)—the carb should be covered.

As most people drink alcohol in the evening—as a before-dinner cocktail, with a meal, or after a meal—you may need to eat a bedtime snack (if you usually don't) or have a bigger snack than you usually do. This is to compensate for the alcohol in your system that is lowering your blood glucose level. Obviously, much depends on whether this is a nightly ritual and you have a good feel for what the alcohol does to your blood glucose and how to compensate with your insulin dosing or whether it's a rare occasion and you are guessing at how your blood glucose might react.

If you have a mixed drink with fruit juice or a carbohydrate-containing beverage, check the amount of carbohydrate in the drink and add it to the total carb in the meal or snack. Then calculate your insulin based on your I:Carb ratio. Checking your blood glucose before and after you drink the alcoholic beverage (and eat the meal), you can get a better idea of its effect on your blood glucose level.

WHAT DO YOU DO WHEN THERE IS A VARIATION IN BLOOD GLUCOSE LEVELS BUT NO SPECIFIC PATTERN?

Look for changes in your daily schedule, such as missed meals or variable amounts of physical activity. These will throw your blood glucose levels off and make you think that your I:Carb ratio isn't working. Check your records, do you find:

▩ Missed meals or snacks	☐ yes	☐ no
▩ Variable activity	☐ yes	☐ no
▩ Stress	☐ yes	☐ no
▩ Varied eating schedule	☐ yes	☐ no
▩ Different amount of carbs	☐ yes	☐ no

If you answer "yes" to several or all of these, then do you also find in your records:

▩ Insulin doses that change often	☐ yes	☐ no
▩ Frequent hypoglycemia	☐ yes	☐ no
▩ Frequent hyperglycemia	☐ yes	☐ no

There is a connection between the changes in the first list and the results in the second list. Let's practice sleuthing. Your fasting blood glucose is in your target range and you are having a pattern of high blood glucose levels related to a specific meal. The meal is usually one you eat at a restaurant or a friend's home or consists of foods that you have not eaten in the past.

Your I:Carb ratio is 1 unit of rapid-acting insulin for every 15 g of carb, and you have a target range of 75 g of carb. You take 5 units to cover the meal based on your I:Carb ratio, but your blood glucose is high after that meal. You could have miscalculated the carbs in the meal. If your estimate of the carbs is off, do a review of weighing and measuring your servings or the contents of the meal to get back on track.

Or let's say you eat out at a favorite restaurant and order a specific item you enjoy and your after-meal blood glucose levels are higher than your target. Record the grams of carb that you estimate in the meal and how many units you took to cover it. After you've had the meal several different times, check your records for how many units of insulin you took to cover the meal and what your blood glucose was after the meal, and you will have a good idea of how much insulin you need to take the next time. Another option is to purchase the meal, take it home, and weigh and measure the contents. Look up the carb content of the ingredients and then total the carb grams. This gives you a number to work with next time you have this meal.

There is no substitute for blood glucose checks and keeping detailed records to sort out the changes in patterns. Discuss the changes and possible causes and solutions with your health care provider.

HOW DOES PHYSICAL ACTIVITY AFFECT YOUR BLOOD GLUCOSE LEVELS?

Physical activity will generally lower blood glucose. So to deal with increased physical activity, reduce your insulin dose or eat more carbohydrate to compensate. Your goal is to prevent hypoglycemia. For safety, always try to have your blood glucose levels between 80 and 180 mg/dl while being physically active. Immediately and several hours after you are active don't let your blood glucose drop below 70 mg/dl. You may need to do blood glucose checks before and after exercise if you are active forty-five minutes or more. If the exercise is long and intense, check your blood glucose over the next twenty-four to thirty-six hours, because it can continue to fall for that length of time.

Balancing blood glucose levels with irregular amounts of physical activity can be challenging. It takes some thinking and planning with insulin and food. Obviously, it's easiest to regularly integrate physical activity into your life. This is the easiest way to learn what it will do to your blood glucose levels and how you need to adjust your food and both your rapid-acting and longer-acting insulin.

Yet another advantage of most insulin pumps with physical activity is that you can at any time decrease the basal rate of insulin. This allows you to get less insulin during the course of the activity and, if needed, a reduced amount of insulin several hours after the activity when your body is utilizing an increased amount of glucose.

Do keep in mind that physical activity doesn't always raise blood glucose. If you have type 1 diabetes and you don't have sufficient insulin in your body at the time you are active, your blood glucose levels can rise. The general rule is to not exercise if your blood glucose level is above 250 mg/dl and you have some ketones. Use this advice if it is early in the day before you have eaten anything, if it is more than three to four hours after a meal, or if you believe you missed your last dose of rapid-acting insulin.

WHAT ABOUT STRESS?

Stress is a normal part of life, but it can interfere with blood glucose control. Your appetite, how well you rest, and how much physical activity you get may all change when you are under stress. Sleep may be inadequate during times of stress. Even though it would be the best thing for you, you may not get enough physical activity to promote relaxation during stressful times. This may be a time that blood glucose levels go up and down unpredictably, and this can be related to not having your regular routine. Stress also interferes with blood glucose control by the release of certain hormones. These hormones can cause your body to release additional glucose into your bloodstream and can also interfere with the action of insulin. This can cause blood glucose levels to be high, and therefore, your insulin requirements can be high, too.

There are many ways that people cope with stress. And different people cope with stress differently. For example, people eat too much or too little, sleep too much or too little, or drink too much. The more you learn your blood glucose's reaction to stress, the better you can do some advanced planning to keep your blood glucose levels in control. There is no way to escape all stress in life. However, if you currently find that stress is causing big problems for you, you might want to learn some healthy coping skills, such as walking, yoga, deep breathing, or listening to soothing music. These may help you keep your blood glucose in better control during these times.

IF I AM INTERESTED IN GOING ON AN INSULIN PUMP, HOW CAN I FIND OUT MORE ABOUT THE PUMPS AND THE REALITIES OF USING A PUMP?

Today, more and more people are choosing to go on an insulin pump. The main reasons are flexibility in managing life and diabetes and improved blood glucose control. You might consider a pump if you:

- Have type 1 diabetes and want more flexibility with insulin and timing of meals

- Have type 2 diabetes and take four shots of insulin a day and want more flexibility

- Have type 1 or 2 diabetes and want to get better blood glucose control

- Have particular problems managing blood glucose levels overnight or with irregular bouts of activity

- Have gastroparesis (a diabetes-related digestion problem)

Today there is no particular age you must be to go on a pump. There are very young children on pumps whose parents do all of the management. There are older people as well. Today many health plans cover part or all of the pump and related supplies. The most important things to do if you are interested in moving to a pump are to:

1) Educate yourself about insulin pump therapy in general (see resources below)
2) Educate yourself about the various features of the different insulin pumps (see web site addresses and toll-free numbers)
3) Find a diabetes care provider who works with insulin pumps and make sure you can have a good partnership with them and their staff

The pumps available today are still so-called "open loop" pumps. They don't have a glucose sensor with an automatic insulin delivery system built in. However, the available pumps keep getting more sophisticated. The current generation of several of the companies' pumps can interact with a blood glucose meter, factor in I:Carb ratios, and even estimate the insulin left "on board" prior to your next bolus.

To find out more about each of the individual pumps, you can go to the companies' web sites. The following is a list of the web-sites for the most popular pumps in the United States. Each of these companies makes one or more insulin pumps. If you become more serious, contact the companies. They will get you in touch with a local sales representative who will be glad to set up an appointment with you to teach you more about the pump as well as the associated costs and medical coverage.

- Animas Corporation: *www.animascorp.com*; 1-877-767-7373

▪ Deltec: *www.delteccozmo.com*; 1-800-826-9703

▪ Disetronic: *www.disetronic-usa.com*; 1-800-280-7801

▪ Medtronic (Minimed): *www.minimed.com*; 1-800-826-2099

(Note several other pumps are available in the U.S.)

To learn more about insulin pumping in general the following are excellent resources:

Smart Pumping, by Howard Wolpert, MD (editor). American Diabetes Association, 2002.

Pumping Insulin, 3rd ed., by John Walsh, PA, and Ruth Roberts, MA. Torrey Pines Press, 2000.

www.insulin-pumpers.org
www.diabetesnet.com

Another resource to consider that is likely available in your area is an insulin pump support group. The sales representatives from the various insulin pump companies will be able to tell you where and when these meet. You don't have to be on a pump to go to one. Attending a support group is a great way to talk to people who have made the decision you are contemplating.

WHERE DO YOU GO FROM HERE?

By now you are probably more comfortable with Carb Counting, but after all this practice there will be times that you find your I:Carb ratio is not quite right and your blood glucose levels are higher than your target ranges. What can you do about it? Always start with the basics. Measure the serving size and the amount of carbohydrate in it. Check your weighing and measuring of foods and see if your portions have grown or shrunk. Review your label reading and interpretation skills and check those for accuracy. Go through your checklist of things in your life that could have changed—your weight, your activity level, your diabetes and other medications. Doing a quick review of these "quality assurance" checks every so often is helpful. Balancing your food, medication, and physical activity to control your blood glucose is and will remain a daily challenge. But hopefully with all this new knowledge and these skills in hand managing diabetes will seem like less guesswork.

15

Cornerstones

Knowledge and Support

You can build good control of your diabetes one experience at a time. It's important to realize that you will constantly be building your database of experiences. To do this, it's helpful to have some help—people around you who can provide you with knowledge and support. That's knowledge to take care of your diabetes day to day and support to keep on keepin' on, even when your motivation is burnt out.

Knowledgeable health care providers can offer education, insights, and resources. They can serve as your coaches and offer support in their role as your cheerleaders. Your family members and friends may also be able to support you and celebrate your progress in meeting the challenges before you. Use a variety of avenues to seek out your coaches and cheerleaders.

Find Your Carb Counting Coach

If you decide Carb Counting is for you, you can begin a hunt for a Carb Counting coach by looking for a registered dietitian (RD) who is also a certified diabetes educator (CDE). This isn't a must, but an RD, CDE, should be able to help you master Basic and Advanced Carbohydrate Counting. How do you find an RD, CDE?

This depends on where you live and how electronically connected you are. Try one or all of the following phone numbers or web sites.

AMERICAN DIABETES ASSOCIATION DIABETES EDUCATION PROGRAMS THAT ARE RECOGNIZED BY ADA

The American Diabetes Association (ADA) has a process for recognizing diabetes education programs that meet certain quality guidelines. Going to one of these programs ensures that you receive quality diabetes education. It also ensures that an RD is part of the program. It is also likely that the RD is a CDE. These programs are located all over the U.S. and usually offer diabetes education group classes and one-to-one counseling. The people who provide the education are usually nurses and dietitians. Some programs may also have exercise physiologists, pharmacists, or behavioral counselors.

Two ways to find these ADA diabetes education programs in your area:

- Call the ADA at 1-800-DIABETES (1-800-342-2383). Ask for the program nearest you.

- On the ADA web site go directly to recognized programs at: *www.diabetes.org/education/eduprogram.asp.*

AMERICAN ASSOCIATION OF DIABETES EDUCATORS

The American Association of Diabetes Educators (AADE) provides you with two routes to find a diabetes educator. AADE is an association of nearly 10,000 health professionals who provide diabetes education. Diabetes educators may be nurses, nurse practitioners, dietitians, exercise physiologists, pharmacists, social workers, behavioral counselors, or psychologists. Diabetes educators are typically found at hospitals providing their services both in the hospital and to outpatients, at managed care organizations, in endocrinologists' offices, in large group-physician practices, at their own independent facilities, and more. Many diabetes educators choose to become a CDE. You will find CDEs at ADA-recognized diabetes education programs (see above).

Two ways to find a diabetes educator:

- Call AADE at 1-800-TEAMUP4 (1-800-832-6874). The person who answers the phone will ask for your zip code and then will give you the names of some diabetes educators in your area.

- On the Internet, go to *www.diabeteseducator.org/Find AnEduc/index.html* and click on the state in which you want to find an educator.

THE YELLOW PAGES

You might find diabetes programs or RDs at your local hospital or listed in the yellow pages. Look up "Endocrinologist" under "Physicians" in the phone book. Call and ask if they know of diabetes education programs or diabetes educators who are dietitians in your area.

TALK TO PEOPLE

Talk to people who have diabetes or people in a diabetes support group to see if they can recommend a health professional.

Do You Know the Questions to Ask?

Once you have the names of a couple of diabetes educators, call and ask them a few questions about their knowledge of and their approach to Carbohydrate Counting. You want to make sure you get what you are looking for. Tell them you want to learn either Basic or Advanced Carbohydrate Counting and why.

- Ask if they teach Carbohydrate Counting and what types.

- Ask about their breadth of experience.

- Ask how many sessions they think it will take for you to master Carb Counting.

- Ask if they provide their teaching only in groups or in groups and individually.

- Ask about the cost of a session or the program.

- Ask whether they bill your health plan or if you must submit the claim to your health care plan.

- Ask whether their services are likely to be covered by your health plan.

Is Diabetes Education and/or Nutrition Counseling Covered by Health Insurance?

For starters, there's no single answer to this question The answer depends on your health coverage and the regulations—either state or federal—that apply to your health coverage. Traditionally, diabetes education (now called diabetes self-management training) and nutrition counseling for diabetes (also referred to as medical nutrition therapy, or MNT) have not been covered by health insurance plans. However, today the odds have improved greatly. That's in part because Medicare now covers some MNT for diabetes and most states have laws on the books to mandate that some health plans cover this service. However, it will be best if you contact your health plan using the toll-free number on your insurance card to get the details about their coverage of diabetes education and MNT for diabetes. Ask about whether the service is covered, the number of visits covered, whether you have to go to a particular person or program, and whether you need a referral for the service from your diabetes care provider.

If you feel you should be covered for diabetes self-management training and/or MNT but your health plan is denying this coverage, then ask questions and demand answers. Plead your case.

If your health plan isn't willing to cover diabetes self-management training and/or medical nutrition therapy or you have no health insurance, then the choice is yours as to whether to reach into your pocket and pay for these services. You are likely to realize it is money well spent. Also, you'll likely realize that—all things considered—a few sessions with a knowledgeable diabetes educator is not that expensive when compared to medications, hospitalizations, or even the cost of a restaurant meal.

Form Your Cheerleading Squad

Beyond the how-to skills and knowledge, you need continuing support when it comes to managing the day-to-day challenges of taking care of diabetes. There will be times that you are gung-ho and feel your Carb Counting efforts are paying off and other times where you just don't see the point in trying to control your blood glucose because nothing you do seems to work. Yes, you need diabetes educators to help you become more knowledgeable, but you also need them to be part of your cheerleading squad. You need to be able to reach out to them when you need a shoulder to cry on, to brainstorm ideas for working out challenges, to solve day-to-day management problems, or to get a pat on the back when you hit your target goals.

Continue to see your educator after you complete your initial training. Perhaps you come in once or twice a year with a list of questions because you want more information about a particular topic, or your life situation has changed (contemplating a pregnancy, going to college, retiring, or other life-changing events), or you are concerned that your diabetes has drifted out of control for a variety of reasons. Another way to stay connected with your diabetes educators is to attend a diabetes support group or an insulin pump support group offered by your diabetes educators. In this environment, you not only get support from your educators, but you also encounter cheerleaders in the other members of the group as well. And you have an opportunity to be a cheerleader too.

How Do You Keep on Keepin' On?

One of the most difficult parts of diabetes is staying motivated to keep doing the daily tasks required to take good care of yourself—counting carbohydrates, checking blood glucose several times a day, making medication decisions, taking the medications, checking your feet, and on and on and on. It is easy to suffer from "diabetes burnout." In his book *Diabetes Burnout* (American Diabetes Association, 1999), William Polonsky, PhD, CDE, emphasizes the importance of getting educated and continuing to be educated about diabetes. He states, "Acquiring knowledge and problem-solving skills can provide you with the hope and confidence that is needed to become a good problem-focused cope-er. Because diabetes knowledge is constantly expanding, it is important to stay informed as well. Diabetes support groups and relevant magazines (such as ADA's *Diabetes Forecast*) are likely to be good resources for you."

So, find your coaches—your diabetes educators, doctors, friends and acquaintances who have diabetes, and family members. Utilize them as you continue to learn, solve problems, or deal with unusual situations. Let these people become members of your cheerleading squad.

Dr. Polonsky ends *Diabetes Burnout* with a quote that we think is also an appropriate end to this book. "The fundamental lesson to remember is that feeling stressed about living with diabetes is normal, feeling at war with diabetes is common, but problematic feelings like these can be conquered. With attention, kindness, and humor, you can overcome diabetes burnout and make peace with diabetes. This is not to suggest that you and diabetes will ever become the best of friends, but you can learn to make room for diabetes in your life. And, as you are certain to discover, this will actually improve the quality, and perhaps even quantity, of your life."

Meet Maddie

Maddie is a 71-year-old retired elementary school math teacher. She has had type 2 diabetes for about sixteen years. She has taken moderately good care of her diabetes. Her A1C levels had been between 8 and 9% over the years, but the last two readings were closer to 9%. Unfortunately, she also discovered that her blood pressure was high enough that she needed a blood pressure medication. In addition, she found out she was spilling a small amount of protein in her urine. Maddie was concerned, frustrated, and feeling down about her diabetes. She felt she did a lot to manage her diabetes day to day, but she continued to have a number of high blood glucose levels each week.

When Maddie was first diagnosed with diabetes, she received some education from her doctor and a dietitian. During a few sessions, the dietitian taught Maddie how to use Basic Carb Counting. Maddie was comfortable with this, however, she soon grew tired of the similarity of her meals and the lack of flexibility in her meal plan.

For many years, Maddie had been taking two types of diabetes pills. She was progressively taking larger doses, until she finally reached the maximum dose of each. Maddie's doctor told her that she really needed to think about starting insulin to control her blood glucose levels. Maddie put her doctor off several times by bargaining for more time to "do better on her meal plan." One day Maddie was reading the health section in the local paper. She saw the announcement of a diabetes support group for people with diabetes who take insulin. Maddie decided to attend the next group. She figured that she might get the true lowdown on insulin from people who take it.

When Maddie introduced herself to the group, she let people know she didn't yet take insulin, but her doctor was recommending that she do so. When the group ended, a woman came over to talk with her. She said that she had been in a similar situation about six months prior, but she finally bit the bullet and started taking one type of insulin called Lantus at night. Then, because that wasn't enough to control her blood glucose levels, she started taking rapid-acting insulin before each of her meals. She said she had been amazed at how easy it was to give herself insulin, how much better she now felt, and how much more in control her blood glucose levels were. The woman noted her A1C had gone from 9.3 to 8.2% in six months. This woman also suggested Maddie go see the dietitian at the local hospital diabetes education program. The woman told Maddie that in three sessions, they taught her to do Advanced Carb Counting. She said now she was able to adjust her mealtime rapid-acting insulin dose based on her blood glucose levels and the amount of carb she planned to eat. The woman noted that she ended up paying for the sessions herself because her health plan would not, but she added it was not that expensive and was well worth it.

Maddie felt she had found a new friend—someone who understood her situation. That made her feel good. She vowed to come back to the group's next meeting. She also promised herself she would wake up the next morning and call her doctor to let her know she was ready to go on insulin and call the dietitian to schedule an appointment. Maddie was feeling a bit more positive about her ability and options to get her blood glucose under control.

1

Carb Counts of Everyday Foods

Starches

(includes breads, cereals, grains, starchy vegetables, crackers, snacks, beans, peas, lentils, and starchy foods prepared with fat)
The average grams of carbohydrate per serving = 15 g
The average calories per serving = 80 (this is not true for foods prepared with fat)

Starches	Serving	Calories	Carb (g)	Fiber (g)
Breads				
Bagel	1/2 (2 oz)	160	30	1
Bread, pumpernickel	1 slice	80	15	2
Bread, rye	1 slice	83	16	2
Bread, white, reduced-calorie	2 slices	96	20	4
Bread, white, French, Italian	1 slice	67	12	1
Bread, whole-wheat	1 slice	70	13	2
Bread sticks	2	82	14	1
English muffin	1/2	67	13	1
Hamburger bun	1/2	61	11	1
Hot dog bun	1/2	61	11	1
Pita bread (6" dia.)	1/2	83	17	1
Raisin bread	1 slice	71	14	1

Starches	Serving	Calories	Carb (g)	Fiber (g)
Roll, plain	1	85	14	1
Tortilla, corn, 6–7"	1	56	12	1
Tortilla, flour, 7–8"	1	114	20	1
Waffle, reduced-fat, 4 1/2" square	1	80	16	1
Cereals, cold				
All Bran	1/2 cup	75	22	10
Bran Buds	1/2 cup	112	33	16
Cheerios	3/4 cup	90	16	2
Cornflakes	3/4 cup	89	20	1
Granola, low-fat	1/2 cup	105	21	2
Grape nuts	1/4 cup	105	24	2
Grapenut flakes	3/4 cup	104	24	3
Kix	3/4 cup	66	14	0
Product 19	3/4 cup	88	20	1
Puffed Rice	1 1/2 cup	90	22	0
Puffed Wheat	1 1/2 cup	76	15	1
Raisin Bran	1/2 cup	85	22	4
Rice Krispies	3/4 cup	71	16	0
Shredded Wheat	1/2 cup	90	20	2
Sugar Frosted Flakes	1/2 cup	67	16	0
Wheaties	3/4 cup	80	18	2
Cereals, cooked				
Cream of rice	1/2 cup	63	14	0
Cream of wheat	1/2 cup	67	14	1
Grits	1/2 cup	73	16	0
Oatmeal	1/2 cup	73	13	2
Whole wheat	1/2 cup	75	17	2

Starches	Serving	Calories	Carb (g)	Fiber (g)
Crackers and Snacks				
Animal crackers	8	89	15	0
Crispbread	2 slices	73	16	3
Graham crackers	3	89	16	1
Matzos	3/4 oz	83	18	1
Melba toast	4 slices	78	15	1
Oyster crackers	24	78	13	0
Popcorn, popped, no fat added	3 cups	92	19	4
Popcorn, microwave, light	3 cups (1/2 bag)	65	11	2
Pretzels, sticks/rings	3/4 oz	80	17	1
Rice cake, regular	2	70	15	1
Rye crisp	3 slices	86	20	2
Tortilla chips, not fried	17	82	18	3
Triscuits, reduced fat	5 wafers	81	15	2
Grains				
Bulgur, cooked	1/2 cup	76	17	4
Cornmeal, dry, degermed	3 Tbsp	97	20	2
Couscous, cooked	1/3 cup	67	14	1
Flour, white	3 Tbsp	87	18	1
Kasha	1/2 cup	91	20	2
Millet, cooked	1/4 cup	72	14	1
Rice, white, long grain, cooked	1/3 cup	69	15	0
Rice, brown, cooked	1/3 cup	72	15	1
Wheat germ, toasted	3 Tbsp	80	10	3

Starches	Serving	Calories	Carb (g)	Fiber (g)
Pasta				
Macaroni, cooked firm	1/2 cup	99	20	1
Noodles, enriched egg, cooked	1/2 cup	106	20	1
Spaghetti, cooked firm	1/2 cup	99	20	1
Dried Beans, Peas, Lentils				
Beans				
Baked	1/3 cup	79	17	4
Garbanzo (chickpeas), cooked	1/2 cup	134	22	4
Kidney, canned	1/2 cup	105	19	4
Kidney, cooked	1/2 cup	112	20	6
Lima	2/3 cup	114	21	8
Lima, canned	2/3 cup	125	23	5
Navy, cooked	1/2 cup	129	24	6
Pinto, cooked	1/2 cup	117	22	7
White, cooked	1/2 cup	126	23	6
Lentils, cooked	1/2 cup	117	20	8
Miso (sodium)	3 Tbsp	106	14	3
Peas, split, cooked	1/2 cup	117	21	8
Peas, black-eyed, cooked	1/2 cup	100	18	6
Starchy Vegetables				
Corn, frozen, cooked	1/2 cup	66	17	2
Corn, whole kernel, vac. pack	1/2 cup	83	20	2
Corn on cob, cooked, medium	1 cob (5 oz)	83	19	2
Corn on cob, frozen, 3"	1 cob	70	14	1
Mixed vegetables with corn	1 cup	80	18	4

Starches	Serving	Calories	Carb (g)	Fiber (g)
Mixed vegetables with pasta	1 cup	80	15	5
Peas, green, canned, drained	1/2 cup	59	11	4
Peas, green, frozen, cooked	1/2 cup	62	11	4
Plantain, cooked slices	1/2 cup	89	24	2
Potato, baked with skin	3 oz	93	22	2
Potato, white, peeled, boiled	3 oz	73	17	2
Potato, mashed, flakes (with milk and fat)	1/2 cup	119	16	2
Squash, winter	1 cup	83	22	7
Potato, sweet, canned, vac. pack, pieces	1/2 cup	92	22	3
Yam, plain	1/2 cup	79	19	2

(sodium) = 400 mg or more of sodium per exchange.

Vegetables

(includes raw, fresh, and canned vegetables and vegetable juices)
The average grams of carbohydrate per serving = 5 g

Vegetables	Serving	Calories	Carb (g)	Fiber (g)
Artichoke, cooked	1/2	30	7	3
Artichoke hearts	1/2 cup	36	7	0
Asparagus, frozen	1/2 cup	23	4	3
Asparagus spears, canned, drained	1/2 cup	23	3	2
Beans (green, wax), canned, drained	1/2 cup	14	3	1
Beans, snap, frozen	1/2 cup	18	4	2
Bean sprouts, raw	1 cup	31	6	2
Beets, canned, sliced, drained	1/2 cup	26	6	2
Broccoli, raw, chopped	1 cup	25	5	3
Broccoli spears, frozen	1/2 cup	26	5	3
Brussels sprouts, frozen, cooked	1/2 cup	33	6	3
Cabbage, cooked	1/2 cup	16	3	2
Cabbage, Chinese, raw	1 cup	12	2	1
Cabbage, green, raw	1 cup	18	4	2
Carrots, canned, drained	1/2 cup	17	4	1
Carrots, cooked	1/2 cup	35	8	3
Carrots, raw	1 cup	47	11	3
Cauliflower, frozen, cooked	1/2 cup	17	3	2
Cauliflower, raw	1 cup	25	5	2
Celery, cooked	1/2 cup	14	3	1
Celery, raw	1 cup	19	4	2

Vegetables	Serving	Calories	Carb (g)	Fiber (g)
Cucumber, raw	1 cup	14	3	1
Eggplant, cooked	1/2 cup	13	3	1
Endive/escarole, raw	1 cup	9	2	2
Greens, cooked				
Collard	1/2 cup	17	4	1
Kale	1/2 cup	21	4	1
Mustard	1/2 cup	10	2	1
Turnip	1/2 cup	14	3	2
Kohlrabi, cooked	1/2 cup	24	6	1
Lettuce, iceberg	1 cup	7	1	1
Mixed vegetables (no corn, peas, pasta)	1/2 cup	20	3	1
Mushrooms, canned, drained	1/2 cup	19	4	2
Mushrooms, fresh, cooked	1/2 cup	21	4	2
Mushrooms, raw	1 cup	18	3	1
Okra, frozen, cooked	1/2 cup	34	8	3
Onions, chopped, cooked	1/2 cup	46	11	2
Onions, raw	1 cup	61	14	3
Onion, green, raw	1 cup	32	7	3
Pea pods, cooked	1/2 cup	34	6	2
Pea pods, raw	1 cup	61	11	4
Pepper, green, cooked	1/2 cup	19	5	1
Pepper, green, raw	1 cup	27	6	2
Pepper, hot green chile, raw	1 cup	60	14	2
Radishes	1 cup	20	4	2
Romaine	1 cup	9	1	1

Vegetables	Serving	Calories	Carb (g)	Fiber (g)
Sauerkraut, canned (sodium)	1/2 cup	22	5	3
Spinach, canned, drained	1/2 cup	25	4	3
Spinach, frozen, cooked	1/2 cup	27	5	3
Spinach, raw	1 cup	12	2	2
Squash, summer, cooked	1/2 cup	18	4	1
Squash, summer, raw	1 cup	26	6	2
Tomatoes, canned, solids and liquids	1/2 cup	24	5	1
Tomatoes, raw	1 cup	38	8	2
Tomato juice (sodium)	1/2 cup	21	5	0
Tomato sauce (sodium)	1/2 cup	37	9	2
Turnips, cooked, cubed	1/2 cup	14	4	2
Vegetable juice (sodium)	1/2 cup	23	6	1
Water chestnuts	1/2 cup	35	9	2
Watercress, raw	1 cup	4	0	0
Zucchini, raw	1 cup	18	4	2
Zucchini squash, sliced, cooked	1/2 cup	14	4	1

(sodium) = 400 mg or more of sodium per exchange.

Fruit

(includes fresh, dried, canned, and frozen fruit; and fruit juices)
The average grams of carbohydrate per serving = 15 g

Fruit	Serving	Calories	Carb (g)	Fiber (g)
Fruit, fresh				
Apple, unpeeled, small	1 (4 oz)	63	16	3
Apricots	4	68	16	3
Banana, small	1 (4 oz)	64	16	2
Blackberries	3/4 cup	56	14	5
Blueberries	3/4 cup	61	15	3
Cantaloupe	1 cup	56	13	1
Cherries, sweet	12 (3 oz)	59	14	2
Cranberries	1 cup	47	12	4
Figs, large	1 1/2	71	18	3
Grapefruit	1/2	51	13	2
Grapes, seedless	17	60	15	1
Honeydew melon	1 cup	59	16	1
Kiwi	1	56	14	3
Mango	1/2 cup	68	18	2
Nectarine	1	67	16	2
Orange	1 (6 1/2 oz)	62	15	3
Papaya	1 cup	55	14	3
Peach, medium	1 (6 oz)	57	15	3
Pear, large	1/2 (4 oz)	59	15	2
Pineapple	3/4 cup	57	14	1
Plums, small	2 (5 oz)	73	17	2
Raspberries, black, red	1 cup	60	14	8
Rhubarb	2 cups	52	11	4
Strawberries	1 1/4 cups	56	13	4

Fruit	Serving	Calories	Carb (g)	Fiber (g)
Tangerine, small	2 (8 oz)	74	19	3
Watermelon, cubed	1 1/4 cups	64	14	1
Fruit, canned or jarred, with some juice				
Applesauce, unsweetened	1/2 cup	52	14	2
Apricots	1/2 cup	60	15	2
Cherries, sweet, juice packed	1/2 cup	68	17	1
Cranberry sauce	1/4 cup	86	22	1
Fruit cocktail, juice packed	1/2 cup	57	15	1
Fruit cocktail	1/2 cup	55	14	1
Grapefruit, juice packed	3/4 cup	69	17	1
Mandarin oranges	3/4 cup	69	18	1
Peaches, juice packed	1/2 cup	55	14	1
Pears, juice packed	1/2 cup	62	16	3
Pineapple, juice packed	1/2 cup	74	20	1
Plums, juice packed	1/2 cup	73	19	1
Pumpkin, solid packed	3/4 cup	59	15	6
Fruit, dried				
Apples, rings	4	63	17	2
Apricots, halves	8	66	17	3
Dates	3	68	18	2
Figs	1 1/2	71	18	3
Fruit snacks, chewy, roll	1	78	18	1
Prunes, uncooked	3	60	16	2
Raisins, dark, seedless	2 Tbsp	54	14	1

Fruit	Serving	Calories	Carb (g)	Fiber (g)
Fruit, frozen, unsweetened				
Blackberries	3/4 cup	73	18	6
Blueberries	3/4 cup	58	14	3
Melon balls	1 cup	57	14	1
Raspberries	1/2 cup	61	15	6
Strawberries	1 1/4 cups	65	17	4
Fruit juices				
Apple juice/cider	1/2 cup	58	15	0
Apricot nectar	1/2 cup	70	17	0
Cranapple juice cocktail	1/3 cup	53	13	0
Cranberry juice cocktail	1/3 cup	48	12	0
Fruit juice bars, 100% juice	1	75	19	0
Grape juice	1/3 cup	51	13	0
Orange juice, fresh	1/2 cup	56	13	0
Orange juice, from frozen	1/2 cup	56	13	0
Pineapple juice, canned	1/2 cup	70	17	0
Prune juice	1/3 cup	60	15	1

Sweets and Sugary Foods

The grams of carbohydrate per serving in this group vary quite a bit.
The fat and calorie content vary quite a bit too.

Sweets	Serving	Calories	Carb (g)	Fiber (g)
Angel food cake	1/12 cake	142	32	0
Brownie, unfrosted	2" sq	115	18	4.5
Cake, unfrosted	2" sq	97	17	3
Cake, frosted	2" sq	175	29	6.5
Cupcake, frosted, small	1	172	28	6
Donut, plain cake	1	198	23	11
Donut, glazed (3 3/4" dia.)	2 oz	245	27	14
Fruit spreads, 100% fruit	1 Tbsp	43	11	0
Gelatin, reg. (Jello)	1/2 cup	80	19	0
Gingersnaps	3	87	16	2
Granola bar	1	133	18	5.5
Granola bar, fat-free	1	140	35	0
Honey	1 Tbsp	64	17	0
Ice cream, light	1/2 cup	100	14	4
Ice cream, fat-free, no sugar added	1/2 cup	90	20	0
Jam or preserves, regular	1 Tbsp	48	13	0
Jelly, regular	1 Tbsp	52	14	0
Pie, fruit, 2 crusts	1/6 pie	290	43	13
Pie, pumpkin or custard	1/8 pie	168	19	8.5
Pudding, regular, low-fat milk	1/2 cup	144	26	2.5

Sweets	Serving	Calories	Carb (g)	Fiber (g)
Pudding, sugar-free, low-fat milk	1/2 cup	90	13	2
Sherbet	1/2 cup	132	29	2
Sorbet	1/2 cup	130	31	0
Sweet roll or Danish	1 (2 1/2 oz)	263	36	11
Syrup, maple, regular	1 Tbsp	52	13	0
Syrup, pancake, light	2 Tbsp	49	13	0
Syrup, pancake, regular	1 Tbsp	57	15	0
Vanilla wafers	5	88	15	3
Yogurt, frozen, fat-free	1/3 cup	60	12	0
Yogurt, frozen, fat-free, no sugar added	1/2 cup	90	18	0

Milk and Yogurt

The average grams of carbohydrate per serving = 12 g

Milks and milk products	Serving	Calories	Carb (g)	Total fat (g)
Nonfat or very low-fat				
Buttermilk, low-fat/fat-free	1 cup	99	12	2
Evaporated fat-free milk	1/2 cup	100	14	0.5
Milk, dry, fat-free	1/3 cup	82	12	0
Milk, fat-free	1 cup	86	12	0.5
Milk, 1%	1 cup	102	12	2.5
Yogurt, nonfat, plain	3/4 cup (6 oz)	90	13	0
Yogurt, nonfat, fruit-flavored, nonnutritive sweetener	1 cup	100	17	0
Low-fat				
Milk, 2%	1 cup	121	12	4.5
Sweet acidophilus milk	1 cup	110	12	3.5
Yogurt, low-fat, plain	3/4 cup (6 oz)	112	13	3
Yogurt, low-fat, with fruit	1 cup	253	47	3
Whole				
Whole milk	1 cup	150	11	8
Evaporated milk	1/2 cup	169	13	10
Goat's milk, whole	1 cup	168	11	10

Meat and Other Foods that Contain Mainly Protein and Fat

Most of the foods in this group—meats, poultry, seafood, eggs—contain no carbohydrate. However, several foods in this food group—processed meats, tofu, cheeses, and peanut butter—contain very small amounts of carbohydrate.

	Serving	Calories	Carb (g)	Total fat (g)
Meat				
Beef, jerky, dried (sodium)	1 oz	94	4	4
Fish sticks (2)		152	13	7
Meat sticks, smoked	1 oz	153	15	14
Tempeh	1/4 cup	83	7	3
Tofu	1/2 cup	94	2	6
Cheese				
Cheese, fat-free	1 oz	37	3	0
Cottage cheese, nonfat	1/4 cup	35	3	0
Ricotta, part-skim	1/4 cup	86	3	5
Processed American cheese, fat-free	3/4 oz slice	30	2	0
Peanut butter, chunky	1 Tbsp	94	4	8
Peanut butter, smooth	1 Tbsp	94	3	8

Fats

Many of the foods in this group–margarine, butter, oils, olives, bacon, and sausage–contain no carbohydrate. Several foods in this food group–nuts, salad dressings, low-fat and fat-free mayonnaise, and spreads–contain very small amounts of carbohydrate.

	Serving	Calories	Carb (g)	Total fat (g)
Nuts				
Almonds	1 oz	165	6	15
Cashews	1 oz	161	9	13
Peanuts	1 oz	165	5	14
Pecans	1 oz	189	5	19
Pumpkin seeds	1 oz	126	15	6
Walnuts	1 oz	182	5	18
Salad dressings				
Salad dressing, fat-free	1 Tbsp	20	5	0
Salad dressing, reduced-fat	2 Tbsp	80	5	6
Salad dressing, regular	1 Tbsp	64	2	6
Mayonnaise				
Mayonnaise, fat-free	1 Tbsp	10	2	0
Mayonnaise, reduced-fat	1 Tbsp	40	3	3

Alcohol

Note: Most of the calories in alcoholic beverages are provided by the alcohol. Most alcoholic beverages contain no carbohydrate, but other beverages do. When you drink alcohol, be careful because alcohol can either make your blood glucose rise or fall too low. See pages 85–87 about the use of alcoholic beverages.

Beverage	Serving	Carb (g)
Beer (regular)	12 oz	13*
Beer (light)	12 oz	5*
Brandy	1 1/2 oz (1 shot)	0
Liquor (any type; for example, gin, rum, vodka)	1 1/2 oz (1 shot)	0
Liqueur (any type, for example, Kahlua, creme de menthe)	1 1/2 oz (1 shot)	14–18*
Wine (white)	4 oz	1*
Wine (red)	4 oz	3*

* These are average numbers. Check the carbohydrate count for the specific alcoholic beverage you choose from a nutrient database. Nutrition Facts labels do not appear on alcoholic beverages.

Carb Counting Resources

Today, due to Nutrition Facts labels, books, and a plethora of Internet resources, there's a ton of carb counts for foods at your fingertips, from the common apple to the more obscure caramola (starfruit) to many foods from a variety of cultures and more. Here's a brief compilation of some of the best and most reliable resources available. A word to the wise—you only need to have a few resources at your fingertips. There is no need to overwhelm yourself, your bookshelves, or your computer.

We've divided these resources into three groups. That's because the foods for which you need carb information fall neatly into the following three groups:

1. Foods that have Nutrition Facts labels
2. Foods that don't have a Nutrition Facts label (such as fresh produce)
3. Restaurant foods

Within this list of resources find the group or groups of foods for which you need information. Then observe the suggested resources for that group of foods and gather what you need.

1. Foods that have a Nutrition Facts label:

If you have a Nutrition Facts label in front of your nose, by all means use it. It's readily available, accurate, and up to date. It's also free. Look under **Serving Size** to determine if the serving you will eat is the same or different. Next observe the **Total Carbohydrate** grams. You can pretty much ignore the **Sugars**. These are already added into the grams of total carbohydrate.

2. **Foods that don't have a Nutrition Facts label:**
   Most of these books contain nutrition information for most foods purchased in a supermarket. They contain information for both foods without Nutrition Facts labels and those with Nutrition Facts labels. Only use these books for the former. Use the Nutrition Facts label if it is in your hand. Some of these books and resources also contain information for restaurant foods. Also remember that as a starting point you have Appendix 1 of this book, which is a list of 500 of the foods Americans most commonly eat.

BOOKS:

- *The Diabetes Carbohydrate and Fat Gram Guide*, 2nd ed., by LeaAnn Holzmeister, RD, CDE. American Diabetes Association, 2000.
  This book provides the carbohydrate count as well as other nutrition information for thousands of foods including fruits, vegetables, and other produce; meats, poultry, and seafood; desserts; many foods you know by their brand name; frozen entrées; and more.

- *The Doctor's Pocket Calorie, Fat and Carbohydrates Counter*, by Allan Borushek. Family Health Publisher, 2004.
  This book provides the calorie, fat, and carbohydrate information for thousands of basic and brand names foods.

- *Calories and Carbohydrates*, 15th ed., by Barbara Kraus. Mass Market Paperback, 2003.
  This book provides the carbohydrate and calorie count for more than 8,000 foods including fruits, vegetables, and other

produce; meats, poultry, and seafood; desserts; many foods you know by their brand name; frozen entrées; and more.

◼ *Bowes and Church Food Values of Portions Commonly Used*, 17th ed., by Janet Pennington. J.P. Lippincott Company, 1998.

◼ *The Corinne T. Netzer Carbohydrate Counter*, 7th ed., by Corinne T. Netzer. Dell Publishing, 2002.
This book provides the carbohydrate count for thousands of foods including fruits, vegetables, and other produce; meats, poultry, and seafood; desserts; many foods you know by their brand name; frozen entrées; and more.

WEB SITES:

◼ *www.nal.usda.gov**
This gets you to the Federal Governments' Nutrient Databases. You can download this database of 6,000 basic foods for free. Go to "Publications and Databases." Click on "Databases." Go down to "USDA Nutrient Databases for Standard Reference." Go to "For more information." Then to "Download." As of October 2002, this database is available online: *www.nal.usda.gov/fnic/foodcomp*

◼ *www.calorieking.com*

◼ *www.nutritiondata.com*

*Note: there are a number of online dieting web sites, such as *ediets.com, weightwatchers.com*, or *caloriescount.com*, that contain nutrient databases. These web sites also often provide you with sample meal plans based on your nutrition needs and preferences. To use most of these you need to become a member. There are also many web sites that allow you to calculate the nutrient composition of the foods you eat. Keep in mind that all these resources use, as their core list of foods, the

USDA database noted above to which you have free access. Therefore, you might as well use the original source.

3. Restaurant foods:

Web sites

- Review chain restaurants' web sites. Many of the large national chain restaurants' web sites provide nutrition information, including information about carbohydrates. For example: *www.mcdonalds.com*, *www.pizzahut.com*, etc. (Very little information is available from sit-down table-service types of chains.) See further explanation and tips for estimating carb counts in chapter 10.

BOOKS:

- *Guide to Healthy Restaurant Eating*, 2nd ed., by Hope Warshaw, MMSc, RD, CDE. American Diabetes Association, 2002.
  This guide provides the basics about today's diabetes nutrition and meal planning, meal-planning goals, and strategies for healthy restaurant eating. Plus, there's nutrition information including carbohydrate, calories, fat, percent of calories as fat, saturated fat, cholesterol, sodium, fiber, and protein with servings or exchanges for more than 3,500 menu items from nearly fifty-five major restaurant chains.

- *Eat Out, Eat Right*, 2nd ed., by Hope Warshaw, MMSc, RD, CDE. Surrey Books, 2003.
  This book contains information about eating healthy in more than twenty types of restaurants, including ethnic cuisines with healthier and not-so-healthy ingredients, cooking methods, and suggested menu items and glossaries of terms for ethnic cuisines. Two sample meals based on healthy eating targets show the reader just how to put healthy meals together, plus hundreds of practical tips and tactics.

▒ *Nutrition in the Fast Lane—The Fast Food Dining Guide.* Franklin Publishing Inc., 2004.

This booklet, which is updated annually, provides the nutrition information for fifty-four of the popular chain restaurants.

SOFTWARE FOR PDAS FOR CARB COUNTS AND/OR DIABETES MANAGEMENT:

▒ ezManager and ezManager Plus from Animas (*www. animascorp.com*). Database of 9000 foods with ability to input insulin-to-carb ratios and activity.

▒ HealthTech.com has several products available, including glucopilot, balancelog, PXNutrition info. Visit at *www.healthetech.com.*

▒ Freestyle Tracker meter, which is a meter with a Visor PDA. Able to track blood glucose readings, insulin, food, and activity. Learn more at *www.therasense.com/tracker* (2500-food database).

(See page 149 in chapter 11 to learn more about the computer-based programs available to track your data.)

Record Keeping Forms

Carbohydrate Counting and Blood Glucose Results Record

Day/Date: _____

Time/ meal	Diabetes medicines		Food		Carb count (servings/ grams)
	Type	**Amount**	**Type**	**Amount**	

Notes about day:

				Blood glucose results			
Fasting/ before b'fast/ time	**After b'fast/ time**	**Before lunch/ time**	**After lunch/ time**	**Before dinner/ time**	**After dinner/ time**	**Before bed/ time**	**Other/ time**

Sample

Carbohydrate Counting and Blood Glucose Results Record

Day/Date: _Tuesday, June 3_

Time/ meal	Diabetes medicines		Food		Carb count (servings/ grams)
	Type	**Amount**	**Type**	**Amount**	
6:45 a.m./ B'fast	H	4 u	Shredded Wheat 'n Bran with Cheerios Milk Banana	1/2 cup 3/4 cup 1 cup 1 large	
12:30 p.m.	H	5 u	Sub sandwich– 12" turkey, ham, cheese, lettuce, tomato, onions, pickles, mustard Pretzels	1 2 1/2 oz bag	
5:00 p.m.			Apple	1 large	
7:15 p.m. Dinner	H	7 u			
10:00 p.m.	Lantus	14 u			

Notes about day:
Went for a walk after dinner. Felt a bit low an hour after return (see other BG).

			Blood glucose results				
Fasting/ before b'fast/ time	**After b'fast/ time**	**Before lunch/ time**	**After lunch/ time**	**Before dinner/ time**	**After dinner/ time**	**Before bed/ time**	**Other/ time**
92/6:30 A.M.	179/ 9:10 A.M.						
		123/ 12:30 P.M.	89/ 2:00 P.M.				

Build Your Food and Carb Counting Database

As you begin to use Carb Counting to control your diabetes, you will find out the carb count of many foods—the crackers you buy, the apples you usually choose, your favorite ice cream, frozen entrée, recipe, or restaurant meal. Rather than having to keep a mental list of the carb counts of these foods or having to look them up every time, start to build your Carb Count Database. This information helps you keep track of the foods, the servings you usually eat, the carb count, and any notes you want to record. For example, maybe you find that a particular food does (or does not) make your blood glucose rise as much as you thought it would or a particular food is a good snack before exercise or on a full day of hiking.

You can keep this record in a notebook, a computer file, or on your handheld day timer. Keep it in a convenient place and in a format that works for you.

Carb Count Database

Food	Serving (amount I eat)	Carb servings/grams	Notes (effect on blood glucose level, what you would do next time you eat this, etc.)

Sample

Food	Serving (amount I eat)	Carb servings/grams	Notes
Bagel (Dunkin' Donuts)—pumpernickel	1	70	More carbs than I thought!
Grandma Grace's Apple Cobbler	3/4 cup	35 (from recipe analysis)	Don't need as much insulin as I thought I would to cover it.
Domino's cheese pizza with onions and mushrooms—hand tossed	2 14" pieces	45	Raises my blood glucose most 3 hours after I eat it.
Healthy Choice Ginger Chicken Hunan	1 entrée	59	Quick rise in blood glucose.
Weight Watcher's Garden Lasagna	1 entrée	30	Works well.

Here's another example of a chart you can use for your database of foods.

Food	My usual serving	Grams of carbohydrate	Notes about effect on BG level	Notes for next time I eat this food/meal

Sample

Food	My usual serving	Grams of carbohydrate	Notes about effect on BG level	Notes for next time I eat this food/meal
Dry cereal, Shredded Wheat 'n Bran mixed with Raisin Bran	1 cup (1/2 cup of each)	59	1 hour after eating— BG 185 2 hours after eating— BG 220	Decrease amount of cereal or take more rapid-acting insulin
McDonald's Quarter Pounder with small fries and 1% milk	1 1 1	37 26 13 ── 76	2 hours after eating— BG 165	Took 5 units of rapid-acting insulin to cover meal— worked well

Index

About the American Diabetes Association

The American Diabetes Association is the nation's leading voluntary health organization supporting diabetes research, information, and advocacy. Its mission is to prevent and cure diabetes and to improve the lives of all people affected by diabetes. The American Diabetes Association is the leading publisher of comprehensive diabetes information. Its huge library of practical and authoritative books for people with diabetes covers every aspect of self-care—cooking and nutrition, fitness, weight control, medications, complications, emotional issues, and general self-care.

To order American Diabetes Association books: Call 1-800-232-6733. http://store.diabetes.org [Note: there is no need to use **www** when typing this particular Web address]

To join the American Diabetes Association: Call 1-800-806-7801. www.diabetes.org/membership

For more information about diabetes or ADA programs and services: Call 1-800-342-2383. E-mail: Customerservice@diabetes.org www.diabetes.org

To locate an ADA/NCQA Recognized Provider of quality diabetes care in your area: Call 1-703-549-1500 ext. 2202. www.diabetes.org/recognition/Physicians/ListAll.asp

To find an ADA Recognized Education Program in your area: Call 1-888-232-0822. www.diabetes.org/recognition/education.asp

To join the fight to increase funding for diabetes research, end discrimination, and improve insurance coverage: Call 1-800-342-2383. www.diabetes.org/advocacy

To find out how you can get involved with the programs in your community: Call 1-800-342-2383. See below for program Web addresses.

- *American Diabetes Month:* Educational activities aimed at those diagnosed with diabetes—month of November. www.diabetes.org/ADM
- *American Diabetes Alert:* Annual public awareness campaign to find the undiagnosed—held the fourth Tuesday in March. www.diabetes.org/alert
- *The Diabetes Assistance & Resources Program (DAR):* diabetes awareness program targeted to the Latino community. www.diabetes.org/DAR
- *African American Program:* diabetes awareness program targeted to the African American community. www.diabetes.org/africanamerican
- *Awakening the Spirit: Pathways to Diabetes Prevention & Control:* diabetes awareness program targeted to the Native American community. www.diabetes.org/awakening

To find out about an important research project regarding type 2 diabetes: www.diabetes.org/ada/research.asp

To obtain information on making a planned gift or charitable bequest: Call 1-888-700-7029. www.diabetes.org/ada/plan.asp

To make a donation or memorial contribution: Call 1-800-342-2383. www.diabetes.org/ada/cont.asp